The Truth About Hormone Replacement Therapy

Scientific Reviewers

Philip A. Corfman, M.D., FACOG
Nancy A. Dreyer, MPH, Ph.D.
Nancy Reame, Ph.D.
Lynn Rosenberg, Sc.D.
Anthony Scialli, M.D.

The Truth About
Hormone
Replacement
Therapy

How to Break Free from the
Medical Myths of Menopause

National Women's Health Network

Cynthia Pearson

Adriane Fugh-Berman, M.D.

Amy Allina

Charlea Massion, M.D.

Mariamne Whatley, Ph.D.

Nancy Worcester, Ph.D.

Jane Zones, Ph.D.

with Ellen Michaud, Contributing Writer and Editor

PRIMA PUBLISHING

Published by Prima Publishing, Roseville, California. Member of the Crown Publishing Group, a division of Random House, Inc.

PRIMA PUBLISHING and colophon are trademarks of Random House, Inc., registered with the United States Patent and Trademark Office.

The information provided in this book is not intended to be a substitute for professional or medical advice. All readers are urged to consult with a doctor or other medical professional before embarking on, modifying or ending any medical treatment.

Library of Congress Cataloging-in-Publication Data on File

ISBN 0-7615-3478-4

02 03 04 05 HH 10 9 8 7 6 5 4 3 2

Printed in the United States of America

First Edition

Visit us online at www.primapublishing.com

Contents

Acknowledgments

This book has grown over the past thirteen years out of the work of the National Women's Health Network, including five previous editions, published by the Network under the name *Taking Hormones and Women's Health: Choices, Risks and Benefits*. Some of the authors listed on this updated and expanded version of the book have been involved since the beginning, and others have joined along the way.

Since the publication of the first edition in 1989, many people have contributed their time and expertise to help make this book accurate, interesting, and useful. We would like to acknowledge the contributions of the following people to previous versions: Davi Birnbaum, Mary Frances Duggan, Denise Fuge, Mary Goodwin, Maxine Jo Grad, Brooke Grandle, Ginger Gregory, Jane Heimlich, Ethel Kahn, Anne Kasper, Miriam Kinman, Laura Kittross, Victoria Leonard, Margie Maddox, Deborah Narrigan, Judy Norsigian, Tracey Orloff, Jennifer Owens, Lori Roseberry, Norma Swenson, Diana Waterhouse, and Louise Wen.

We also want to acknowledge the tens of thousands of people who have been members of the Network over those years. These women and men see the need for independent information about hormone replacement therapy and, with their support, have made the Network's efforts in this area possible.

Finally, we would like to thank the founders of the Network—Phyllis Chesler, Belita Cowan, Mary Howell, Barbara Seaman, and Alice Wolfson—who did the groundbreaking work that provided access to information about the risks and benefits of birth control pills and hormones used around the time of menopause.

About the Authors

The National Women's Health Network

Founded in 1975, the National Women's Health Network is the only national membership organization devoted solely to the health of all women. The mission of the Network is to advocate for national policies that protect and promote all women's health and to provide evidence-based, independent information to empower women to make fully informed health decisions.

To accomplish this mission, the Network:

- Acts as an independent voice for women's health and thus accepts no money from companies that sell pharmaceuticals, medical devices, dietary supplements, alcohol, tobacco, or health insurance;
- Represents and is supported by individual and organizational members;
- Researches and analyzes women's health issues from a feminist, critical perspective free from the influence of corporate interests;
- Creates and disseminates evidence-based information on women's health issues to consumers, advocates, health care professionals, media, and policy makers;

- Monitors and educates Congress and federal agencies to ensure that laws and policies as well as research and regulatory decision-making reflect the interests of all women;
- Monitors information provided by companies that sell or promote pharmaceuticals, medical devices, and dietary supplements;
- Links activists and community groups nationwide;
- Addresses the interconnections among health and social, racial, economic, and gender equity.

Cynthia Pearson

Cindy Pearson is the executive director of the National Women's Health Network. In addition to representing the Network in the media and to the government, Ms. Pearson has served on the boards of the Reproductive Health Technologies Project, the National Breast Cancer Coalition, the Campaign for Women's Health, the D.C. Women's Council on AIDS, and the National Action Plan on Breast Cancer, as well as the advisory board of the Boston Women's Health Book Collective. Ms. Pearson has received the Special Service Award from the National Association for Women's Health, the Commissioner's Special Citation from the Food and Drug Administration, and the Margaret Sanger Award from the Federation of Feminist Women's Health Centers. She has also received recognition of her contribution to women's equality and human rights from the Feminist Majority Foundation.

Prior to working at the Network, Ms. Pearson served as the director of Colorado NARAL and Womancare Clinic in San Diego, California.

Adriane Fugh-Berman, M.D.

Adriane Fugh-Berman is assistant clinical professor in the department of health care sciences at George Washington School of Medicine. She is editor of the CME newsletter, "Alternative Therapies in Women's Health" (American Health Consultants, Atlanta), and author of *The 5-Minute Clinical Consult to Herbs and Dietary Supplements* (Lippincott, Williams and Wilkins, 2002) and *Alternative Medicine: What Works* (Lippincott, Williams and Wilkins, 1997). She consults on dietary supplements and herbs for the Federal Trade Commission and is a member of the Institute of Medicine Committee on Establishing a Framework for Evaluating Dietary Supplements and U.S. Pharmacopoeia's Expert Committee on Dietary Supplements. From 1995 to 1998, Dr. Fugh-Berman was a medical officer at the Contraception and Reproductive Health Branch, NICHD, NIH. Prior to that, she worked in the Office of Alternative Medicine, NIH. Dr. Fugh-Berman is a board member of the National Women's Health Network and writes on women's health issues for *Natural Health* magazine. A graduate of Georgetown University School of Medicine, Dr. Fugh-Berman's post-graduate training was in the family practice track of the Residency Program in Social Medicine, Montefiore Medical Center, Bronx, New York. Dr. Fugh-Berman's articles have appeared in the *Lancet, Psychosomatic Medicine, Journal of*

Nervous and Mental Disorders, Preventive Cardiology, and other medical and consumer publications. She has appeared on the *Today Show, Nightline,* and *20/20.*

Amy Allina

Amy Allina is the program and policy director of the National Women's Health Network. She plans and implements the Network's policy agenda on a range of issues, including menopause, reproductive health, access to health care, and regulation of drugs and devices for women. She represents the organization with government agencies, legislative bodies, and the media. Prior to joining the Network in 1999, Ms. Allina worked on women's health policy issues at the consulting firm of Bass and Howes and as the political organizer for the Maryland affiliate of NARAL. Ms. Allina also served as Associate Editor of *Multinational Monitor,* a monthly magazine founded by Ralph Nader, and is a member of the board of directors of My Sister's Place, a shelter for battered women and their children in Washington, DC.

Charlea Massion, M.D.

Charlea Massion is a board-certified family physician and a women's health specialist who practices at the Santa Cruz Medical Clinic in Aptos, California. Dr. Massion is on the clinical faculty in the division of family and community medicine at Stanford University School of Medicine, is on the editorial advisory board of Alternative Therapies in Women's Health, and is a founding board member of the American College of Women's Health

Physicians. Dr. Massion studies physician-patient communication issues and leads seminars in physician health and career development.

Mariamne H. Whatley, Ph.D.

Mariamne H. Whatley, a biologist, is Evjue-Bascom Professor of Women's Studies, chair of the women's studies program, associate dean in the school of education, and professor of curriculum and instruction at the University of Wisconsin-Madison, where she has been teaching women's health since 1978. Her research focuses primarily on women's health and on sexuality education. She recently co-authored, with Elissa R. Henken, *Did You Hear About the Girl Who . . .? Contemporary Legends, Folklore, and Human Sexuality.*

Nancy Worcester, Ph.D.

Nancy Worcester is an associate professor in women's studies and continuing studies at the University of Wisconsin-Madison. In this position, she regularly teaches a science-based women's health course on campus to four hundred students a semester, coordinates and teaches a wide range of women's studies courses off campus, and developed, coordinates, and is the key trainer for the Domestic Violence Training Project. Dr. Worcester has a Ph.D. in nutrition from the University of London. She developed women's studies programming in the 1970s in England while working as a head of department at a large adult education center (Richmond Adult College). She has been a women's health writer, organizer, and lecturer for thirty years, being a founding member of the National (Britain) Women's Health Information Center and serving on the National (USA) Women's Health Network board of directors for twelve years. Dr. Worcester is the co-editor, with Mariamne H. Whatley, of three editions of *Women's Health: Readings on Social, Economic, and Political Issues.*

Jane Sprague Zones, Ph.D.

Jane Zones is a medical sociologist in the department of social and behavioral sciences at the University of California, San Francisco. An advocate for women's health for more than thirty years, teaching courses in women's health and policy since 1975, she has published a variety of articles in the area, particularly on drug and device technology and regulation. Dr. Zones chairs the California Women's Health Council and the Board of Breast Cancer Action, and is a member of the advisory board of the California Women's Health Collaborative. She is a past chair of the board of the National Women's Health Network, and has been a member of several scientific advisory panels of the Food and Drug Administration, most recently the Reproductive Health Drugs Advisory Committee.

Ellen Michaud

Ellen Michaud, contributing writer and editor, is *Prevention* magazine's editor-at-large. She is the author of numerous health books, including *Total Health for Women* and *The Healing Kitchen.*

Introduction

The widespread popularity of hormone replacement therapy in the United States is a triumph of marketing over science and advertising over common sense. As a society, we ignore the fact that menopause is not a disease. It is a normal transition that occurs in all women.

Many consumers (and their health care providers!) honestly believe that hormone replacement therapy (HRT, the use of estrogen together with progestogen) or estrogen replacement therapy (ERT, the use of estrogen alone) prevents a variety of serious diseases and helps women look younger.

Despite this belief, there is no valid scientific evidence that estrogen prevents heart disease, colon cancer, Alzheimer's disease, or wrinkles. What the evidence does show is that estrogen reduces some symptoms of the menopause transition. Women should be aware that there are other choices for dealing with these symptoms.

No randomized, placebo-controlled trial to date has shown that hormones prevent heart disease. Claims to the contrary are based on old, scientifically flawed observational studies whose results cannot be trusted. This is why the Food and Drug Administration (FDA) has never approved any form of estrogen for heart disease prevention. For more information, see chapter 14 "The Studies," and appendix A.

What's more, evidence gathered from studies on the benefits of HRT in preventing colon cancer, Alzheimer's, and wrinkles is inconclusive and conflicting. In the past few years, for example, several studies reported that women taking ERT and HRT were less likely to develop or die from colon cancer.[i, ii, iii] However, like other supposed benefits claimed in observational studies, the fact that healthier women chose to take hormones in the first place may account for the apparent risk reduction.

As for osteoporosis, there is good evidence that estrogen delays bone loss for as long as a woman takes it, but the evidence that it reduces fractures when they are most likely to happen—around age eighty—is weak. In fact, studies show that taking measures to prevent falls lowers fracture risk far more than any drug can. Unfortunately, this fact does not stop the osteoporosis industry from exaggerating the likelihood of fractures and disability and bombarding consumers with advertisements for HRT and ERT.

Confusing the picture even more is a new category of drugs known as Selective Estrogen Receptor Modulators (SERMs). These drugs are the "designer estrogens" we frequently hear about. SERMs purportedly give us the alleged benefits of hormone therapy without the risks. However, the long-term safety and efficacy of these drugs has not been demonstrated.

When Is HRT a Good Idea?

Scientific evidence supports the use of HRT only in the following cases:

- for women who have had both ovaries surgically removed at an early age
- for women with severe hot flashes, night sweats, or vaginal dryness
- as one option for maintaining bone density in women at high risk of osteoporosis

For women who experience troublesome hot flashes or vaginal dryness, we recommend they try nonhormonal therapies as the first line of treatment. Later, if a woman chooses hormones, we suggest she take the lowest dose for as short a time as possible.

There really is no easy answer to the conundrum should I or shouldn't I take hormones. However, women need to know that scientific evidence does not support

---

HRT Has Not Been Shown To

- Prevent wrinkles or other natural signs of aging
- Cure urinary incontinence
- Help moodiness or depression
- Improve sexual desire or responsiveness
- Prevent heart disease
- Improve memory
- Prevent Alzheimer's disease

---

routine use of hormones in menopausal or perimenopausal women. What's more, it is poor public health practice to attempt to prevent chronic diseases by recommending drugs of unknown efficacy and known adverse effects to an entire population, when lifestyle measures or other therapies may achieve the same or better benefits.

One simple remedy is exercise. Regular exercise protects bones, reduces the risk of falls, reduces the risk of heart disease, and increases the sense of well-being. Except for an occasional strain or sprain, sensible, regular exercise has no negative side effects.

Many women who go ahead and use HRT experience higher rates of blood clots and possibly breast cancer. They are more likely to undergo hysterectomies or have their gallbladders removed. Taking hormones also makes mammograms more difficult to read so that HRT users are more likely to get false mammogram readings and miss the diagnosis of breast cancer in its earliest, most treatable stage.

The Bottom Line

To us, the bottom line is clear. Some health care providers who have not done their homework are pressuring women to take hormones up to five years before menopause on the theory that hormones support bone health, a notion unsupported by scientific fact. The popular media have jumped on the bandwagon and are urging menopausal women to begin taking hormones as soon as possible.

Both groups make it sound as though the cessation of normal menstrual cycles does lasting harm to the body within days or weeks of its onset. The truth is that it doesn't. Most women have months or years to make decisions about whether or not hormones make sense for them and to reevaluate their decisions as their situations change or as new scientific information becomes available.

It's also important to understand that the risk-benefit calculation for individual women is different at different ages. For most women who start HRT at menopause, the risks come at younger ages, while the benefits emerge much later in life.

On behalf of the entire National Women's Health Network, we urge you to take all the time you need to make an informed decision about starting or continuing hormones. Read this book, paying particular attention to the studies listed in chapter 14. Also, talk to your health care provider and think about all the issues involved until you feel you know the truth about HRT.

We hope that this book serves as a sensible guide to help you make the best possible decision for you.

PART ONE

Why This Book Is Needed

CHAPTER ONE

Manufacturing Need, Manufacturing Knowledge

Pharmaceutical companies spend big bucks and use inventively camouflaged strategies to manipulate you and your health care provider.

When it comes to menopause, the flood of unreliable information is a major problem for women and their health care providers. Pharmaceutical companies influence almost everything we know about menopause, including our decisions about treatment. Recent questions about the accuracy of drug ads in general only heighten the confusion.

Even savvy consumers are usually unaware of the many ways that their health care providers are pressured into thinking that menopause is a disease requiring medical treatment. Practitioners themselves often don't realize how their "education" on menopause and menopausal products has been deliberately manipulated by the drug companies, whose first priority is to sell these products. Nor are health care providers necessarily aware of how artful the drug companies are in manipulating them.

At a recent dinner, a physician commented on how surprised she was to hear that research was beginning to raise questions about whether estrogen really prevents heart disease. Ten years ago, as a medical student, she was a women's health activist and prided herself on critiquing the medicalization of menopause. During the past ten years, however, she became a busy physician and found herself relying on women's health conferences, which were sponsored by the drug industry, for the latest information on menopause. The consistency of the messages she received at these supposedly neutral conferences convinced her to prescribe estrogen to many of her patients, believing she was helping them prevent heart disease. Now she began to wonder if this was so.

> Pharmaceutical companies spend from $8,000 to $13,000 per physician annually to affect drug-prescribing practices.

Pharmaceutical companies spend $8,000–$13,000 per physician annually to affect drug-prescribing practices. Gifts to physicians in training include lunches, books, and stethoscopes. Physicians in practice receive more discreet offerings, such as free attendance at conferences and expenses-paid trips to meetings.

Physicians' acceptance of this cozy relationship is high. Although 85 percent of medical students believe it is improper for politicians to accept gifts from lobbyists, only 46 percent believe it is improper for medical students to accept gifts from pharmaceutical companies.[1]

Yes, There Is a Free Lunch

There are many creative ways that drug companies beguile physicians and other health care providers. The familiar sight of drug company representatives in physician offices is similar to a slew of salespeople selling cosmetics, Fuller brushes, or vacuum cleaners on a homemaker's doorstep every day.

In an office of five physicians, for example, it is likely that there will be four or five drug salespeople a day in patient care areas and the physicians' private offices. The materials they leave in their wake include drug samples; articles from medical journals that support the use of their products; office supplies; food for all medical center staff; small gifts such as clocks, paperweights, mugs, Post-it notes, prescription pads, and candy; and "patient education material" in attractive displays. Even if a physician's policy is not to meet with salespeople, she or he must spend valuable time fending them off every day.

Accuracy is not the drug reps' strong suit. In exchange for a short presentation on their wares, pharmaceutical representatives often bring in lunch for medical students and residents at training hospitals, which increases attendance. A study of the information given during these presentations found that 11 percent of it was inaccurate.[2]

Drug advertisements directed at health care providers are even worse. An assessment of 109 ads in leading medical journals found that the information on efficacy and side effects/contraindications was unbalanced 40 percent of the time. Fifty-seven percent of the ads were judged to have little or no educational value, even though defenders claim the ads provide needed health education.[3]

> An assessment of 109 ads in leading medical journals found that the information on efficacy and side effects/contraindications was unbalanced 40 percent of the time.

Not only physicians are being romanced by drug companies. Nurses, midwives, pharmacists, physician assistants, and nurse practitioners are also wooed. Drug company representatives help these groups fund their professional conferences, give them free publications, bring them meals, and so forth.

This intense daily sales pitch does not occur in other professional workplaces. Architects, for example, do not have to deal with manufacturers of building supplies invading their offices on a daily basis with samples, studies, and presents.

So Little Time, So Many Drugs

Drug company gifts and perks help to build a physician's brand loyalty. Consider the case of Joanne, who was bothered by hot flashes and went to a university medical center to get an estrogen prescription. Because of her involvement with an animal rights group, Joanne told the young doctor who saw her that if her only choice was Premarin (made from the urine of mares who are kept confined and pregnant), she would rather live with the hot flashes. Although there were at least three other estrogen drugs on the market at the time, the young doctor didn't know of even one other drug to give her. Finally, an older doctor stepped in and gave her a prescription for Menest, a plant-based estrogen product.

How does this happen? How does a doctor trained in the most advanced medical system in the world stay so ignorant?

Busy health care providers find themselves surrounded by brand names, and, being human, they succumb. When a health care provider uses a pen advertising drug X to write a prescription on a pad that has ads for drug X inserted between the pages, or sips coffee out of a drug X mug, or scribbles notes on pads and Post-it notes with drug X bannered across the top, and then carries home a clock advertising drug X in a tote bag embossed with the drug X logo, it is no wonder that he or she cannot recall the names of any other drugs.

As one researcher pointed out in a letter to *Lancet*, "No drug company gives away its shareholders' money in an act of disinterested generosity."[4] If these tactics didn't result in selling more drugs and increasing investment returns, you can bet that shareholders wouldn't allow company executives to continue them. Aggressively keeping the company name in front of health care providers sells product.

As for generic equivalents of the high-priced drugs, they are certainly available, as knowledgeable consumers know. They are as good as brand name drugs and quite a bit cheaper, but many doctors just don't know enough about them. Generic drug manufacturers don't have battalions of representatives to invade physician offices, as the brand-name manufacturers do, nor can they compete with the big advertising budgets of brand-name companies. One study found that only 63 percent of family physicians recognized the generic names of ten commonly prescribed drugs, and only 27 percent prescribed mostly generics for their patients.[5]

This ignorance on the part of health care providers costs consumers money. In a study of 1,603 primary care physicians in Kentucky, physicians who relied on information provided by drug reps prescribed more expensive drugs.[6]

How Drug Companies Trick Your Health Care Provider

While outright gifts to health care practitioners are obvious examples of corporate influence, there are other less visible means of affecting medical information that may have far more damaging effects on our health. Here are some.

Medical Conferences

Most health care providers receive their continuing medical education through attendance at medical conference lectures. Unfortunately, drug companies fund much of the information provided at these sessions, often indirectly through a so-called "independent" conference group. Health care providers may know a drug company is "underwriting" a conference or session, but they generally don't realize that some of the lectures embedded within the program are sponsor-produced. The unbiased lectures in the rest of the program deceive health care providers into thinking the entire program is legitimate. Noncommercial talks serve as camouflage for commercial talks.

Informational Materials

Health care providers who give lectures receive very slick prepackaged slide shows, videos, posters, and other glossy materials that they can use in their lectures to other physicians and to their communities. These materials are so fancy that some people joke that you can tell a drug company presentation because the quality of the material is so good (nonprofit groups tend to create graphically challenged overheads via their office computers).

Journals

There are academic journals containing authentic, peer-reviewed articles, and then there are look-alike pseudo-journals put out by drug companies. Physicians read both kinds. Both disseminate drug company propaganda.

As soon as physicians complete their medical training, they start receiving complimentary subscriptions to the reputable *Journal of the American Medical Association* (JAMA) and the *New England Journal of Medicine* (NEJM) from drug companies. They also receive journals published by the drug companies, and it is not always obvious that these journals are not independent. Using the same technique employed at medical conferences, the pseudojournals intersperse objective articles with articles promoting the drug company's products. In contrast with authors of publications in academic journals, who receive no fee, authors of articles in pseudojournals are paid (sadly, sometimes well-known researchers are paid only for the use of their names on articles). The mixture of academic, independent, peer-reviewed journals with fake journals makes it difficult for the practicing physician to distinguish between objective information in the one and cleverly designed advertisement in the other.

A recent study of eight journals published by leading medical organizations found that the estimated amount of money from pharmaceutical advertising ranged from $715,000 to $18 million per year.

Even peer-reviewed journals receive a significant portion of their income from drug company advertising and, therefore, are not immune to drug company influence. In fact, several journals, including the NEJM, have a policy of accepting advertising only for health care products or services.[7] This means that almost all the ads in these journals come from the drug industry.

A recent study of eight journals published by leading medical organizations found that the estimated amount of money from pharmaceutical advertising ranged from $715,000 to $18 million per year. In fact, five organizations raised more than 10 percent of their gross income from one single journal's pharmaceutical advertising. Four raised an equal or greater amount of money from pharmaceutical advertising than from their members.[8]

Research Studies

Pharmaceutical companies influence the topics of medical studies by almost exclusively funding research that boosts their products. For instance, companies that sell osteoporosis drugs are not likely to fund a study that determines whether daily walking builds bone strength. What's more, drug companies may selectively publish only the results that favor their products from studies they have conducted or from studies they funded in which they, rather than the investigators, controlled the data.

Unfortunately, pharmaceutical company funding is easier and faster to attain than federal funding. As a result, much of the research at academic institutions is, in fact, funded by the drug industry. Some researchers sign contracts with gag clauses giving the drug company approval power over manuscripts prior to submission and the option not to publish the study at all. As a result, studies published in the medical literature represent only a fraction of the total number of studies actually conducted.

Because drug companies are not required to publish studies on their proprietary products, no one knows how many drug company–funded studies never see the light of day. However, there's one thing you can count on with studies published by drug companies: They're much more likely to find advantages for a new drug over a standard therapy than are studies funded by other sources.[9, 10, 11]

Bias may also come from scientists who write commentaries or reviews of published research in journals or other professional publications. The investigators of a study that assessed seventy articles on blood pressure medications contacted the authors of the articles to ask about any financial relationships they may have had with manufacturers.[12] They found that *96 percent of those who wrote articles favorable to a drug had financial relationships with the manufacturer,* as compared with 37 percent of authors who stated unfavorable results. Another study that examined forty-four articles on the cost-effectiveness of six oncology drugs found that only 5 percent of studies funded by pharmaceutical companies reported negative results, compared with 38 percent of studies funded by nonprofit entities.[13]

The bottom line?

Drug companies influence the information that health care practitioners receive through selective study funding, selective study publication, pseudojournals, drug company–funded conferences, personal visits from gift-bearing representatives, and supposedly objective medical conference lectures. Much of this influence is subtle, insidious, and often inaccurate. Nevertheless, drug companies are very effective at convincing health care providers to prescribe expensive, brand-name drugs.

How Drug Companies Trick Consumers

When you open up your Sunday *Parade* magazine and read in the cover story that supermodel Lauren Hutton calls estrogen her favorite beauty secret, do you ever think she might be a paid spokesperson for the Wyeth-Ayerst drug company?[14, 15] Not only is it startling to find that out, but, in fact, it is also just one example of the ways drug companies spend money to influence consumer opinions about their products.

Ads, company-sponsored educational materials, company-initiated "news" stories, company-funded Web sites, and funding of health advocacy and education groups are all strategies the companies use in promotional campaigns designed to sell drugs to consumers. They are parts of a coordinated effort, and they complement similar campaigns targeted at health care providers. The idea behind all these ads, brochures, and news stories is to make sure consumers know the supposed benefits a company's drug has to offer so they will request or accept it when they see their health care providers.

Unfortunately, what these strategies make sure you never learn is anything at all about the risks, the alternatives to the drugs, or the fact that in many cases you don't need to take a drug at all.

Madison Avenue Molds Your Mind

Unless you're completely isolated from the popular media, you've noticed that ads for prescription drugs, including those recommended for menopause, are everywhere these days. Drug ads have become increasingly common since 1997, when the FDA liberalized the rules for advertising on television. Since that change, spending on direct-to-consumer advertising has skyrocketed. In

1999 alone, the pharmaceutical industry spent more than $1.8 billion on direct-to-consumer advertising.[16]

Companies spend this kind of money on ad campaigns because they work. A study by *Prevention* magazine found that one-third of consumers who had seen direct-to-consumer advertisements went on to speak with their health care providers about the medicine advertised,[17] while another study published in a medical journal found that 15 percent of patients would consider switching physicians if their doctor refused a request for a prescription medication they had seen advertised.[18]

Since 1997, spending on direct-to-consumer advertising has skyrocketed. In 1999 alone, the pharmaceutical industry spent more than $1.8 billion on direct-to-consumer advertising.

Drug companies and people who defend the practice of direct-to-consumer advertising say this new trend is good for consumers because it gives them an additional source of information. Yet there are serious drawbacks when consumers make decisions based on information from a source that has a financial stake in their decision.

Take for example a widely published ad by Wyeth-Ayerst promoting the benefits of estrogen. It shows an image of a woman's body and describes evidence supporting estrogen use. It highlights eight body parts and health concerns related to menopause: the brain, hot flashes, sexuality, eyes, teeth, heart, bone, and colon. It doesn't tell us that for five out of those eight indications the benefits of estrogen are not proven. Wyeth-Ayerst has paid the smartest minds on Madison Avenue to come up with the most clever and effective ways to present their product in a positive light, yet no independent authority has reviewed this ad for truthfulness.

Friends on the Take

The ads are reinforced by educational campaigns that appear to be independent but are paid for by the drug companies. These companies seek out nonprofit groups working on women's health and offer them money to conduct educational campaigns that promote the need for their products. These nonprofit organizations produce and distribute educational materials under their own names, and consumers can't tell who wrote the text, much less who paid for it. In one case, the Coalition of Labor Union Women produced a series of fact sheets on women's health paid for by Eli Lilly. The fact sheets covered such issues as cancer, osteoporosis, heart attacks, and menopause.[19] It's surely no coincidence that Evista, which is produced by Eli Lilly but which was not mentioned on the sheets, had potential uses for all of those health problems.

Sometimes, these fact sheets are accurate and well balanced, but sometimes they simply rehash the company's advertisements. The really insidious part is that these materials make it look as though a group that consumers think is independent is raising the health issue out of genuine concern for women, not that some pharmaceutical company is promoting a product and making a profit. This is a particularly pernicious strategy because it undermines consumer trust in legitimate groups working for the public interest. It's also a pervasive strategy. The National Women's Health Network (NWHN) did a study and found that fifteen out of forty-five women's groups had accepted money from pharmaceutical companies.[20]

News You Can't Use

Drug companies are working to influence every source of consumer health information including the actual news. In addition to press releases and press conferences announcing the results of new studies or the launch of new products, companies also produce ready-to-use "news" stories in the form of videos and sample articles and send them to television and radio stations, newspapers, and magazines to broadcast or print directly.

This tactic is very effective. Every single one of more than one hundred television news stations surveyed in one study had used some part of a company-prepared video news release.[21] While responsible journalists will not use these materials without putting them into the context of a fuller story, they are still using the company's materials (and the product name) in their news presentations and putting them into the minds of viewers and readers. When Pfizer launched Viagra, more than 210 million viewers saw some part of the company's video news release.[22]

Even when reporters decide on their own that a new study is worth covering as news, they don't always do a good job of covering the story in a way that's useful for women. Taking the company's promotional materials at face value, they present beneficial findings in the most positive light and downplay or ignore entirely the potential risks. A study that reviewed seventy news stories about positive new findings associated with Merck's drug Fosamax found that barely 50 percent mentioned adverse effects, 70 percent quoted experts or studies with financial ties to the company, and only a third of those pointed out to the viewer or reader the financial ties.[23]

In fact, reporters rarely disclose the financial ties of the physicians and researchers whom they cite as experts on medical matters. Sometimes, those ties create clear conflicts of interest that can affect the accuracy of the medical information the expert is providing for the story.

Web Sites: Partnerships in Deceit?

Like other information sources, Web sites are often subject to influence by corporate marketing. Organizations like Hadassah, the National Council of Women's Organizations, and the Alliance for Aging Research, for example, all carry materials on their Web sites paid for by a grant from Eli Lilly. Disguised as a campaign called the "Partnership for Prevention," these materials look like straightforward health education on menopause, heart disease, and osteoporosis.

They are not. In fact, the information is slanted to motivate postmenopausal women to seek drug treatment. As the Hadassah Web site stated in February 2001, "The risk for heart disease, cancer, and osteoporosis plummets if a woman . . . receives the benefits of estrogen, either naturally or through supplementation."[24]

The placement of marketing information on the Web sites of groups women trust is an insidious tactic. Women need to be aware that information on the Web may be just as biased as any other—perhaps more so because in some cases procedures for regulatory oversight are not yet established.

How to Identify Reliable Information

Is all information tainted? No, there is reliable information out there. However, it can be tricky figuring out which is tainted and which isn't. Here are some guidelines to help:

- **Look for the "virgins."** A common approach in verifying the objectivity of medical information is to turn to a nonprofit organization and see what they have to say. The trouble is, as we have seen, many of the larger nonprofits frequently depend on donations from interested industries. Corporations make donations to nonprofits as an indirect way to market their products. It's not always easy to find out who funds the nonprofits, but often corporation annual reports show who the major donors are, if not the size of their contributions. Also, the Urban Institute's National Center for Charitable Statistics has a Web site (www.urban.org/centers/cnp.html#nccs) that contains financial information about many larger U.S. nonprofits, including a copy of the contributions form that they must send annually to the Internal Revenue Service.

The National Women's Health Network has been called "the only virgin at the orgy" for its policy against taking drug company money.

The Network is not the only "virgin," but the list of others is short. Other nonprofits that we know that have adopted a no-drug-money policy include the Boston Women's Health Book Collective (authors of the best selling *Our Bodies, Ourselves* and *Ourselves Growing Older*), Breast Cancer Action, the Center for Medical Consumers, DES Action, and Public Citizen's Health Research Group.

Consumers do well to seek out these groups, which develop and distribute reliable and science-based information on women's health, as well as maintaining informational Web sites. When individuals join and contribute to these organizations, they help the groups keep their independence.

- **Follow the money.** Check the funding sources of any organization that provides health-related information. Many seemingly neutral and objective pamphlets and brochures given out free at health fairs or in health providers' waiting rooms are funded with drug company money. Look for a small, two-line attribution to the company at the bottom of the back page.

- **Notice sources of bias in the public sphere.** Newspapers, magazines, Web sites and other media are more dependent for their income on advertisers than they are on subscribers. Not only the ads but also information included or not included in the actual content of most media are strongly affected by who their advertisers are. One of the better-known examples of this in the past was the lack of information about tobacco's effects on health in women's magazines that accepted cigarette ads.

- **Read the research yourself.** It's easy to locate current research using the National Libraries of Medicine database called MEDLINE. It is available online at www.nlm.nih.gov/databases/freemedl.html and through local libraries.

> Many seemingly neutral, objective pamphlets given out for free at health fairs or in waiting rooms are funded with drug company money.

You don't have to be a doctor to understand and raise questions about medical research. Virtually all studies follow a similar format. First, read the abstract, the brief summary at the beginning of the article, to see if the article addresses your concerns. The discussion section at the end often gives a context for interpreting the study findings, and this is also where a good research report will discuss its own limitations.

Also near the end of an article (though at times up front) in the more respected medical journals is an author's statement of conflict of interest. This statement should include sources of funding for the research. Generally (though not always), funding from public sources, such as the National Institutes of Health, indicates independence from companies that have a financial interest in the results of the study. If the funder is an organization you haven't heard of, it might be a good idea to look on the Internet to see if it has industry ties. University research centers often provide grants that may seem "clean," for example, but you need to be aware that some universities get substantial funds from private groups with conflicts of interest. If there is industry funding for a study, you need

> University research centers often provide grants that may seem "clean," but be aware that some universities get substantial funds from private groups with conflicts of interest.

to find out whether the money came with strings attached: Did the investigators have independent control over the data and publication decisions, or did the company play a role in determining what was done with the research results?

See appendix A for a quick course in research analysis. With this information, you can evaluate how close a study comes to being free of commercial interest. Near the end of a semester-long college women's health course, for instance, one of the students asked, "If none of us is a scientist, and we can figure out what's wrong with these studies, why can't the doctors?" The answer is that doctors can figure it out, but they usually don't have the time to read and analyze all the research they see. Fortunately, concerned consumers and advocacy groups can take the initiative to figure out the truth on their own.

CHAPTER TWO

Estrogen Forever?

A chronology of one of the most successful prescription drugs in the United States

"Hot flashes making you uncomfortable?"

"Night sweats ruining your sleep?"

"Hair sprouting on your chin?"

"Alligator skin turning you into a piece of old leather?"

If you answered yes to any of these questions during a doctor's appointment in 1965, chances are that your family physician nodded wisely, pulled out a prescription pad, and told you to take estrogen.

That's because pharmaceutical companies of that era, aided and abetted by many popular media, were aggressively promoting estrogen as an anti-aging drug,

Animal Rights Activists Oppose Premarin

The most visible opponents of HRT are not women's health groups but animal rights groups who have exposed the cruelty to mares involved in the production of Premarin. An estimated 75,000 pregnant mares are used to produce Premarin and related products. The constantly pregnant mares are kept in small stalls, and their slaughtered foals have become a $9-million-per-year industry as a delicacy in Belgium, France, and Japan. Animal rights groups estimate that Wyeth-Ayerst will use one less pregnant mare for every 150 women who decide not to take Premarin.[3]

even though the medical evidence supporing some of these claims was just as weak or weaker then as it is today.

Feminine Forever by Dr. Robert A. Wilson, a consultant to the manufacturers of Premarin, egged them on.[1] Wilson's book promoted estrogen as a wonder drug that allowed women to age more slowly, look more attractive, and avoid the up, down, and sideways mood swings that popular wisdom said accompanied the "change of life."[2]

Premarin is a drug made by forcing pregnant (PRE) mares (MAR) to spend their lives tethered in small stalls attached to urine (IN) collection devices. By 1975, as a result of Wilson's book, Premarin was one of the five most prescribed drugs in the United States.[4]

The Big Shock: Estrogen and Endometrial Cancer

In December 1975, women who took estrogen learned to their dismay that two studies linked estrogen to endometrial cancer. The studies concluded that women taking estrogen were *five* to *fourteen* times more likely to develop endometrial cancer than women who weren't taking it.[5, 6]

The National Women's Health Network, whose founders had earlier alerted women to the risks of oral contraceptives, organized a demonstration at the Food and Drug Administration, calling for informational patient package inserts (PPIs) for all estrogen products. The FDA complied. However, in 1977, the American College of Obstetricians and Gynecologists and others sued the FDA to block the package inserts.

Premarin is a drug made by forcing pregnant (PRE) mares (MAR) to spend their lives tethered in small stalls attached to urine (IN) collection devices.

The FDA, with the NWHN and other consumer organizations as codefendants, won the court case, and thereafter PPIs for estrogen products became a permanent FDA requirement.[7] Also in 1977, Network cofounder Barbara Seaman published a landmark book, *Women and the Crisis in Sex Hormones.*

The PPIs and extensive media coverage of estrogen's cancer risks led to a dramatic drop in estrogen prescriptions.[8] In 1979, in what seemed the coup de grace for ERT, a Consensus Conference at the National Institutes of

Health rejected almost all claims for the physical and psychological benefits of ERT. The conference committee—a blue ribbon panel of doctors and researchers from around the country—concluded that estrogen was only effective in alleviating hot flashes and vaginal dryness.

Combined Hormone Therapy

During the 1980s, preliminary epidemiology studies demonstrated that the increased risk in uterine cancer associated with estrogen was diminished by combining estrogen with a progestogen.[9] Drug companies, loathe to lose the large market of menopausal women, began a publicity campaign and gradually convinced clinicians that lower doses of estrogen combined with progestogens eliminated the risks of estrogen taken alone.[10] The mixture was dubbed "Hormone Replacement Therapy" (HRT). It was a successful campaign: By 1988, a significant shift in prescription patterns had taken place.[11]

> In 1979, a Consensus Conference at the National Institutes of Health rejected almost all the claims for the physical and psychological benefits of ERT.

Marketing Fear: Estrogen and Osteoporosis

In the early 1980s, the Ayerst company (now Wyeth-Ayerst), manufacturer of Premarin, funded a public relations campaign that included "educational" efforts by the Nursing Association of the American College of Obstetricians and Gynecologists.[12] The campaign attempted to link menopause and osteoporosis—even though bone loss occurs in men as well as women, starting in the fourth decade of life.

When a 1984 National Institutes of Health (NIH) Consensus Conference reviewed studies (conducted only in white women) and concluded that estrogen delayed postmenopausal bone loss and reduced the number of hip and wrist fractures, the pharmaceutical industry ran with it.[13] By the late 1980s, CIBA, manufacturer of Estraderm, was running ads that pictured older women with dowager's humps. The scary ads encouraged women to ask their doctors about estrogen to prevent osteoporosis.[14]

In 1986, the National Osteoporosis Foundation was created with drug company support. This group continues to overstate the number of women who will experience the most debilitating effects of osteoporosis—even though studies show that most women with the disease do not experience the severe problems that women fear.

Widening the Market:
Estrogen and Heart Disease

By the late 1980s, several studies had found that women who'd had heart attacks were less likely to have used estrogen than women who had not.[15] So, in 1990, Wyeth-Ayerst asked the FDA to approve Premarin as a preventative for heart disease in postmenopausal women.

The evidence was much weaker than that usually required for approval of a new drug intended for long-term use in healthy people, and the FDA refused. Despite this rejection, clinicians routinely recommended that menopausal women take estrogen to prevent heart disease.[16] In 1989, the American Heart Association held a conference on women and heart disease emphasizing the alleged protective effects of estrogen.

The Nurses Health Study: Estrogen and Breast Cancer

In 1990, a report from the Nurses Health Study, the largest women's health study in the United States to date, found a *36 percent* greater chance of women with breast cancer having used estrogen than women without cancer.[17]

Soon after, the federal Centers for Disease Control and Prevention (CDC) published a summary analyzing sixteen separate studies, again linking hormone use to a 30 percent increase in breast cancer.[18]

> In 1990, a report from the Nurses Health Study found a 36 percent chance of women with breast cancer having used estrogen than women without cancer.

Unfortunately, the exposure of estrogen's down side did not appear to be as newsworthy as its benefits: The *New York Times* ran the article on the heart disease benefits of estrogen on page one, while the article linking estrogen to breast cancer ran on page eighteen.[19, 20] Carol Ann Rinzler's book, *Estrogen and Breast Cancer,* also met with media silence.[21] Scrupulously researched and documented, with a foreword by respected Harvard researcher Graham Colditz, the book received few reviews in the mainstream press.[22]

The Women's Health Initiative

In September 1993, the NIH began the first large, long-term study on the safety and effectiveness of ERT and HRT. (This study—the Women's Health Initiative—also looks at the roles of calcium, vitamin D, and low-fat diets.)

Twenty-five thousand postmenopausal women ages fifty to seventy-nine from diverse ethnic groups were assigned at random to take ERT, HRT, or a placebo for nine years. They are being monitored for heart disease, cancer, osteoporosis, and cognitive function (including dementia). We strongly support the study, which will answer many questions about HRT and ERT use. The first results will be announced sometime in the year 2005.

Heart Moves Center Stage

In April 2000 and then again in 2001, preliminary findings from the still-in-progress Women's Health Initiative indicated *significantly higher* risks (*not* benefits) of heart disease in the first few years of the trial in women who take either ERT or HRT, compared with women who do not. While it's necessary to continue the trial to find out whether these results will hold up, they do cast new doubt on the theory that taking hormones can prevent heart disease.

Preliminary findings from the Women's Health Initiative indicated *significantly higher* risks (*not* benefits) of heart disease in the first few years of the trial in women who take either ERT or HRT.

Also in 2001, the American Heart Association issued a science advisory recommending that women with heart disease should not begin HRT and clearly stating that there is not enough evidence to support starting a woman on HRT solely to prevent heart disease.

History Repeats Itself

At the same time as alleged heart benefits are being called into question, we are experiencing a resurgence of "fountain of youth" claims for estrogen. Like Dr. Robert Wilson in *Feminine Forever*, the new generation of estrogen enthusiasts claim that estrogen use will give women more supple skin, better moods, better memory, and sharper concentration.[23] These claims play on women's fear of aging—particularly the fear of dementia and disabilities—and they emphasize a possible role for estrogen in preventing Alzheimer's disease. Although these claims are not supported by conclusive scientific evidence, they have received much media hype. After many years leading the list, Premarin has been surpassed, but it is still the second biggest selling drug in the United States.

It is not a coincidence that we focus so much attention on menopausal and aging issues, including "quick fix" pharmaceutical solutions for osteoporosis and heart disease. Since more funding became available for women's health research, there has been a new emphasis on such disease-specific studies. Besides diverting focus from broader approaches to women's health, these studies have largely excluded the analysis of the social and political contexts of disease prevention that was the hallmark of women's health movements in earlier years.[24]

Then, in the 1990s, "baby boomers" reached midlife. More women in this age group than ever before have good jobs and "disposable" income, thus expanding the potential profit a company can make from these consumers. As a result, menopause issues have become commercialized and mainstreamed, with many marketing specialists promoting products (sometimes entire catalogues of products!) to female baby boomers and their health care providers.

Women may seem to have access to a lot of information with which to evaluate these products, but the range of viewpoints and options is limited by the parameters of profit. Marketers do not get paid to promote nonprofit products or information, so midlife women are more likely to see an ad for beautifully and expensively packaged vaginal weights to prevent bladder prolapse or increase orgasm than to see a well-produced leaflet on how and why simple, do-it-yourself vaginal exercises (or Kegel exercises) are important. Similarly, midlife women will find much more information on hormones and drugs than lifestyle-centered health promotion. Disease prevention information rarely addresses the wider social, economic, and political realities of women's lives.

Women who are skeptical of the medicalization of menopause and who do not jump on the Premarin band-wagon are also targets of advertisers. Small and large companies market so-called "natural" hormones or "alternative" products to these women, even though there is little evidence supporting the efficacy or safety of medicinal herbs to treat menopausal symptoms.

CHAPTER THREE

Menopause, Natural and Not

Each woman experiences menopause differently.

When Martha Correll hit age forty-two, her life got complicated. "Let's just say I had PMS, cramps, periods, hot flashes, insomnia, and a toddler," she says now. "It was a really hot summer, and at first I thought it was just the weather that was bothering me. I'd hang out with other moms at our kids' playgroup, and the heat just drove us crazy."

After talking with her older sister who's a nurse, Martha realized that her hot flashes and resulting insomnia meant that her body was getting ready for menopause, a natural process that every one of us will experience if we live long enough with our ovaries intact. By contrast, Rosalyn Reich breezed through her menopause. "I think I had a hot flash once," she says. "It happened when I thought I had lost a chapter of my dissertation."

During the reproductive years, our ovaries are the main producers of estrogens and progesterone and at relatively high levels. During the years leading up to menopause (the "perimenopause"), ovarian production of estrogen and progesterone begins to fluctuate, and ovulation and bleeding patterns change and become irregular.

Different women have different rates and patterns in their menstruation, which may explain variations in how they experience menopause.

Eventually, the ovaries almost stop producing estrogen altogether. Estrogen and progesterone levels drop below the minimum needed to continue menstrual cycles, and menopause—literally defined as the cessation of menstruation—occurs. Different women have different rates and patterns, which may explain the variations in how they experience menopause. With Martha, for example, it began at age forty-two—the same age as her mother and sister before her. Among Martha's friends, changes began anywhere from age thirty-eight to fifty-one.

The Ups and Downs of Menopause

Although we often hear that ovarian estrogen production declines in a straight line, hormone levels actually fluctuate quite a bit. Some of the changes associated with perimenopause are the result of high, rather than low, levels of hormones as well as rapidly changing levels. An abrupt drop in estrogen levels is almost certainly associated with a more sudden onset of menopausal "symptoms," while a gradual drop usually accompanies a gradual appearance of symptoms.

Most "Perimenopausal Symptoms" Also Affect Men

If you think that symptoms like dizziness, headaches, tiredness, nervousness, aggressiveness, irritability, incontinence, joint pains, palpitations, insomnia, and listlessness are part of menopause, you're right.

You're also wrong.

Turns out that although all these symptoms affect women during the perimenopausal years, many of them affect men as well. A Dutch survey of 8,679 men and women over age twenty-five found, for example, that except for the excessive sweating typical of hot flashes and night sweats, men had exactly the same complaints as women of the same age.

There's just no evidence that symptoms other than hot flashes and night sweats are either gender or age specific. The researchers concluded that a hormonal cause of these complaints, therefore, seems unlikely."[1]

After menopause, the ovaries continue to produce low levels of estrogens and androgens. The adrenal glands—small glands located above the kidneys—also produce both hormones. Androgens are also converted to estrogen by fat tissue.[2]

Contrary to the popular description of ovaries dying and postmenopausal women having no estrogen, women continue to produce roughly 10 percent of their former estrogen after menopause and throughout the rest of their lives.

Where You Live Makes a Difference

The hormonal changes that accompany menopause vary among individual women and among cultures. Some women breeze through menopause, while others experience heavy and unpredictable bleeding, painful intercourse, and hot flashes that disrupt sleep.

Women whose menopause is induced by surgery, chemotherapy, or other medical treatment in which ovarian hormone synthesis stops suddenly often have more severe symptoms. Cultural conditions also play a role, with the incidence and type of symptoms varying widely in different parts of the world.

Research done on Japanese women, for instance, reveals a low rate of hot flashes and few menopausal complaints.[3] In contrast, Greek women are more likely to experience hot flashes, although they don't seek medical care for them. Mayan women, whose diet and lifestyle are very different from women in industrialized countries, look forward to menopause and do not report any hot flashes or other bothersome changes.[4]

> Contrary to the popular description of ovaries dying and postmenopausal women having no estrogen, women continue to produce roughly 10 percent of their former estrogen after menopause and throughout the rest of their lives.

While women in Europe and North America associate menopause with hot flashes, night sweats, irritability, and depression, women in northern Thailand associate menopause with headaches, and

Menopausal Myths

Myth 1: *Menopause causes osteoporosis, heart disease, arthritis, and other chronic diseases.* False! Menopause does not cause these or any other chronic conditions. Just because certain ailments and menopause all happen on the way to getting old doesn't mean one causes the other.

Myth 2: *Menopause causes mood changes.* Nope. Many of the psychosocial changes attributed to menopause occur just as frequently in women in other age groups. And guess what? Men report almost all the same symptoms as women, thus the notion of "male menopause." It's not menopause that causes mood changes—it's life!

Myth 3: *Menopausal women are estrogen deficient.* Wrong again. Postmenopausal women continue to make estrogen from their ovaries and their adrenal glands. In fact, postmenopausal women with ovaries are no more "estrogen deficient" than prepubertal girls—each has an appropriate level of estrogen for her phase of life.

Myth 4: *In the old days, women didn't use to live past menopause; modern women live longer and thus need estrogen.* No way! Decreased infant and maternal mortality mean more women live to ripe old age, but hundreds of years ago, women who survived childhood diseases and dangerous childbirth practices also lived long lives!

Japanese women associate it with shoulder stiffness and headaches, but not hot flashes or depression.[5] About half of all U.S. women experiencing natural menopause complain of hot flashes.[6] In Japan, approximately 15 percent of women report hot flashes and 3 percent report night sweats.[7]

A Scottish survey of eight thousand women aged forty-five to fifty-four found that 57 percent experienced one or more of fifteen symptoms commonly associated with menopause, but only 22 percent of these found such symptoms a problem.[8] The women reported suffering hot flashes, night sweats, sleep problems, dry/sore vagina, painful joints, headaches, sore breasts, nighttime urination, palpitations, dizziness, irritability, memory problems, anxiety, depression, and feeling unable to cope. Hot flashes and vaginal dryness or soreness were the only symptoms the women associated with menopausal status. Women with surgically or medically induced menopause and HRT users were more apt to report problem symptoms.

Social and Medical Fads Have an Effect on Menopause

It's difficult to determine the importance of cultural factors. Variations in symptoms in different countries could be a result of diet, lifestyle, genetics, or many other factors. However, the fact that Asians respect age while Westerners worship youth makes it hard to escape the notion that menopause in the West might be very different if older women looked forward to an honored place in society rather than discrimination and, in many cases, poverty.

In fact, women's experience of menopause depends in part on the way a society views menopause and aging women. During the era in this country when women were thought to be ruled by their hormones and thus were inferior to men, menopause was a shameful secret. Many women were embarrassed to admit they were undergoing menopause or to seek advice for menopausal discomforts. As late as the 1960s, male physicians described menopause as the end of a woman's active life.[9] Symptoms of aging such as wrinkled skin and memory loss are still falsely believed to be side effects of menopause.

The modern women's movement has changed these old perceptions. Today, much more information about menopause is available, and women now feel comfortable openly discussing the experience. Although some clinicians mistakenly dismiss all physical problems experienced by midlife women as "just" menopause, many are beginning to take women's reports of uncomfortable menopausal changes seriously enough to offer remedies.

The current fashion is for clinicians to treat menopause as a risk factor for long-term diseases, particularly osteoporosis and heart disease.[10] Clinicians also see menopause as a cause of mood changes and mental problems.

> The current fashion is for clinicians to treat menopause as a risk factor for long-term diseases, particularly osteoporosis and heart disease.

Ignoring the fact that postmenopausal women continue to make estrogen, doctors inaccurately describe them as estrogen deficient and tell them that, since estrogen is essential for bodily function, it needs to be replaced.

Particularly misleading is the fact that some physicians take blood samples and then diagnose "low" hormone levels in women whose hormone levels would be low for a twenty-year-old but are perfectly normal for their age. The results are then used to justify treatment that isn't really needed.

Some experts from the old school claim that nature never intended women to live past menopause. They point to the fifty-year life expectancy common at the early part of the twentieth century and allege that modern medicine has kept women alive past their natural lifespans and that a "natural" approach to menopause will not succeed in keeping postmenopausal women healthy. These experts are trying to justify treating menopause as a disease. They have taken menopause, a perfectly normal phase of a woman's life, and "medicalized" it.

Medicalized menopause is not useful to women. Postmenopausal women who have their ovaries are no more estrogen deficient than prepubertal girls. Even in the past, many women lived to a ripe old age. Just look at how our great grandmothers survived childhood diseases and dangerous childbirth practices and lived well into their eighties.[11] Natural menopause does not "cause" osteoporosis or heart disease, conditions that don't usually affect women until twenty to thirty years after menopause.

Surgically Induced Menopause

Unlike the social and medical fads that combine with cultural myths to determine how most women experience menopause, a hysterectomy alters the natural course of menopause altogether. This is because four out of every ten women under age forty-five and seven out of ten older women who have hysterectomies in the United States have their ovaries removed along with their uterus.[12]

The medical name for surgical removal of the ovaries is oophorectomy. Normally, postmenopausal ovaries continue to produce some estrogen throughout life. After an oophorectomy, the absence of the ovaries often causes severe menopausal symptoms that do not respond to natural remedies. Although not conclusive, some studies indicate an oophorectomy may increase your risk of heart disease and osteoporosis.[13] Oophorectomy does lower your risk for breast cancer.

Close to half of all women who had hysterectomies in the late 1980s and early 1990s had both ovaries removed during the procedure.[14, 15] Removing the ovaries is necessary when uterine cancer is present or to treat severe endometriosis. However, many doctors tell women the reason they should have their ovaries removed is to prevent ovarian cancer.

Does This Make Sense?

Women in the United States are three times more likely to have a hysterectomy than are women in Great Britain.[16] What's more, 90 percent of the hysterectomies doctors perform in the United States are for conditions that are not life threatening and could potentially be treated by other means.[17, 18]

We disagree with doctors who practice prophylactic oophorectomy in this context, because ovarian cancer is relatively rare and women need the hormones supplied by their ovaries—even postmenopausal ovaries. Should your physician recommend a prophylactic oophorectomy, we suggest you seek a second or even a third opinion.

This issue of prophylactic oophorectomy is more difficult for women who have a family history of ovarian cancer or who have mutations in genes linked to ovarian and breast cancer. The risk of developing ovarian cancer ranges from 7 percent for women with two affected family members to possibly as great as 50 percent for women who have a family history of several women diagnosed with ovarian cancer at a young age in two or more generations.[19] The risk of ovarian cancer for women with a mutation in breast cancer genes is not yet known, but estimates range from 16 to 44 percent.[20]

For these women, several respected researchers recommend preventative removal of the ovaries by age thirty-five, although this procedure isn't completely effective because some ovarian cells remain.[21, 22, 23, 24]

When Hormone Replacement Is Necessary

We support the use of estrogen by women whose ovaries are removed before age forty-five. In this context, ERT is truly "replacement" therapy, although we emphasize that no pill can replace all of the various hormones lost by surgical removal of the ovaries, nor mimic accurately the delicate interaction among several hormones.

We recognize that some self-help and alternative-medicine activists believe that women who have the willpower to make significant lifestyle changes can produce enough estrogen naturally to avoid the risks typically associated with early removal of the ovaries. Also, some women who are otherwise at low risk for osteoporosis and heart disease may decide not to take hormones after an oophorectomy.

We don't know enough yet about the long-term health issues for women in this situation who choose not to take estrogen.

Medically Induced Menopause

Some premenopausal women lose ovarian function after they have had cancer treatment. Chemotherapy for breast cancer (the most common cancer affecting women under age fifty) often disrupts ovarian hormones. In fact, disrupting ovarian function may be one mechanism by which chemotherapy works. After chemotherapy, women in their thirties often resume normal menstrual cycles. Women in their forties are likely to experience premature menopause.[25]

Radiation used to treat other types of cancer can also bring an end to menstrual cycles.

Currently, premenopausal women facing breast and other cancers have no alternative to treatments that threaten ovarian function. That's why breast cancer activist groups like the National Breast Cancer Coalition have called for research into different types of treatment for cancer.

In the meantime, concern over the long-term effects of medically induced, premature menopause has led to proposals to treat breast cancer survivors with ERT/HRT in order to prevent osteoporosis and heart disease.[26] Short-term studies have begun on this issue, but until long-term results are in, we urge caution. We are concerned that breast cancer survivors who take estrogen may have a higher risk of recurrence of their cancer. (See page 71 for more information about breast cancer survivors and HRT.)

CHAPTER FOUR

The Risks of Hormone Replacement Therapy

HRT gets rid of hot flashes and vaginal dryness. It also increases your chance of developing other health problems.

When Pam Lawson started to go through menopause, she simply wasn't prepared for how little information was available. She went to her health care provider, and he recommended that she go on HRT. She asked if there was anything else she could do, but he implied that she was being silly to worry and said there was nothing wrong with taking hormones. It wasn't until Pam had been taking HRT for several years that she discovered hormones could cause cancer. "I felt so angry and betrayed," she says. "It's my body. I have a right to know the facts before I start taking any treatment. But no one seemed to care or listen. I was treated like a child."

Nine Risks You May Not Want to Take

From their beginnings, ERT and HRT have been controversial. A major part of the problem, as we have said, is the lack of solid information women have to make wise choices. Most of what we know about ERT and HRT comes from women who chose to use the drugs and who agreed to participate in observational studies. These are not controlled studies in which one group is randomly assigned to take a drug and another not to take the drug or to take a different drug. Although controlled studies are the gold standard of modern medicine, there are few on hormone therapy. And most controlled trials are too short to give much useful information about harmful outcomes.

The health problems that appeared in the observational studies have not been proven conclusively to be caused by hormones. To give you the best possible overview of hormone therapy's risks, we've gathered all the studies available, analyzed them, and come up with a list of risks probably—or definitely—associated with the use of estrogen, or estrogen combined with a progestogen. Here's what we've found.

Hormone Therapy May Increase Your Risk of Breast Cancer

Many factors in women's reproductive lives, such as their age when their periods started and when they reached menopause, influence their likelihood of developing breast cancer. Similarly, it seems that taking estrogen also influences the risk of breast cancer.[1]

A few years ago, a welcome summary of nearly every study of estrogen replacement therapy and breast cancer was published. Looking at the experience of more than 52,000 women in 21 countries, the researchers found that women who used ERT for five or more years increased their risk of breast cancer by about 35 percent.[2] The risk lasts as long as a woman takes hormones (and may increase somewhat with even longer use), but disappears within five years after she stops hormone use.

What would happen to younger women if they didn't take hormones and just continued to menstruate?

Because the researchers had access to so much data, they were able to compare risks. They found that each additional year of menstruation increased the risk of breast cancer by 2.8 percent, while each year of ERT/ HRT increased the risk by 2.3 percent.

Not much difference, is there? The similar level of risk adds strength to the conclusion that ERT may in some way promote breast cancer.

Unfortunately, it's unusual for women to hear such a clear and definitive description of the relationship between ERT and breast cancer. Instead, we often hear messages from our clinicians that imply there are only a few studies that have found any risk of breast cancer and dozens that have found no increased risk at all.[3]

These messages are misleading. They ignore the crucially important issue of how long a woman has taken hormones. Although many studies have found no increased risk of breast cancer in women who have "ever" used ERT, the problem with these studies is that women who have "ever" used ERT are likely to have used it for a relatively short period of time. Using ERT for three to five years or less doesn't appear to increase the risk of breast cancer, but using it for five years or longer clearly does.

Unfortunately, the risk of death from breast cancer associated with hormone therapy is less clear, because studies that look at this issue present conflicting results.

The Nurses Health Study's most recent follow-up found a 43 percent increased risk of death due to breast cancer after ten years of hormone use,[4] and a smaller study by researcher Bruce Ettinger and others in California found an increased risk of 89 percent after an average of eighteen years' use.[5] On the other hand, a very large study conducted by the American Cancer Society found that women who reported "ever" using estrogen when they were interviewed in 1982 were 16 percent less likely to die of breast cancer during the next ten years than were women who hadn't used ERT/HRT.[6]

> Using ERT for three to five years or less doesn't appear to increase the risk of breast cancer, but using it for five years or longer clearly does.

Not until 2000 had we had much data on the effect of progestins added to ERT on breast cancer risk. In the past, physicians hoped that progestins would have the same beneficial effect on the breast as they have on the uterine lining and lower any increased cancer risk caused by estrogens alone.

This argument never made biological sense, because progestins and progesterone slow cell division in the uterus, while in the breast they increase it.

Early studies looking at HRT users seemed to show progestins didn't lower the risk of breast cancer.[7, 8, 9] These studies weren't taken very seriously by the average clinician, in part because they involved only small numbers of women. Then, in the year 2000, two large studies confirmed the earlier reports and demonstrated that progestins seem to increase breast cancer risk beyond that of ERT taken alone.[10, 11] As in women who used ERT alone, it seems to take five years before risk increases. After that, the risk increases slightly with each additional year on HRT.

Some women want to know whether the risks of HRT are greater for women who have an inherited risk of breast cancer. Despite this widespread concern, there is only one study specific to this topic. Conducted in Iowa and published in 1997, it is an observational study with inherent weaknesses, but it did follow a large group of women. It found that women with a family history of breast cancer who took HRT were no more likely to get breast cancer than women with a family history who did not take HRT. While one observational study is not definitive, we believe women with a family history of breast cancer probably don't need to worry about the breast cancer risk of HRT any more than women in general.

Hormone Therapy Increases Your Risk of Endometrial Cancer

According to a summary of all studies on endometrial cancer, women who use estrogen alone from one to five years are twice as likely to develop uterine cancer as are

HRT Affects Mammography Readings

Mammography is less effective as a screening tool in women who use hormone therapy.

Several studies have shown that women on ERT or HRT are more likely to have breasts that appear more dense on mammograms.[12, 13, 14] Moreover, recent studies show clearly that ERT/HRT is the cause of increased breast tissue density.[15, 16]

Radiologically dense breasts are a problem because they make it more difficult to detect small breast cancers with mammography. What's more, follow-up studies have shown that mammography is less reliable in hormone users. Not only does hormone therapy make it more difficult to detect early breast cancers, but it also more likely leads to false alarms.

One research group estimated that ERT users are nearly twice as likely to have a biopsy in twenty years of screening than nonusers.[17] This same study found that mammography was also more likely to miss breast cancer in women on ERT/HRT, although the number of cancer cases was too small to make reliable estimates.

Further research is underway to clarify the mammography situation. In the meantime, women who use hormone therapy should be especially attentive to any changes in their breasts, particularly changes that take place only in one breast.

women who have never used hormones.[18] The risk increases to about tenfold after about ten years of use.

The risk depends on the dosage and the number of years that estrogen is taken. Three years of exposure to estrogen in the Postmenopausal Estrogen/Progestin Intervention (PEPI) trial, a national study of nearly nine hundred women, caused abnormal endometrial changes in 34 percent of the women with a uterus.[19] Six percent of the women had to undergo hysterectomies during the study.

Progestogens reduce the risk of endometrial cancer by countering the effects of continuous estrogen, and women who use HRT have a lower risk of endometrial cancer than women on estrogen alone. However, it is still unclear whether women who use HRT have the same or slightly higher risk as women who have never used hormones. All studies have found that taking estrogen and progestin together every day does not increase the risk of endometrial cancer. One study even found that continuous HRT decreased the risk of endometrial cancer to lower levels than women not taking HRT, but it looked at only nine cases. For women who take progestins only part of the month (called sequential HRT), it appears that there is still some increased risk of endometrial cancer. To lower that risk, studies show it is important to take progestins for at least ten days a month.[20, 21, 22, 23, 24, 25, 26]

> All studies have found that taking estrogen and progestin together every day does not increase the risk of endometrial cancer.

The PEPI trial found that every type of progestogen tested protected against precancerous changes in the lining of the uterus. Some clinicians have experimented with progestogens every three months, but a randomized trial testing this strategy using a high dose of estrogen was stopped early after too many women developed troublesome endometrial changes. This approach isn't recommended until more is known.[27]

Hormone Therapy May Increase Your Risk of Ovarian Cancer

ERT and HRT appear to increase the risk of developing ovarian cancer, but, as we noted, the connection between hormone therapy and this cancer has not been confirmed by large, randomized trials. Nine observational studies have looked at the association between ERT/HRT and ovarian cancer. Using ERT/HRT seems to raise the risk of ovarian cancer slightly, and staying on hormones for ten or more years may increase risk by about 30 percent.[28]

Ovarian cancer currently occurs in about one in every fifty-seven women.

Hormone Therapy May Increase Your Risk of Gallbladder Disease

Estrogens in pill form go first to the liver before diffusing into the body's general circulation. A high concentration of estrogen in the liver induces a variety of metabolic processes, including some that are associated with gallbladder disease.

Long-term oral contraceptive users have experienced an increase in benign and malignant liver tumors,[29] although women who take ERT—which contains a different form and dosage of estrogen—have not.

Side Effects

Women sometimes experience the following side effects from estrogen and progestogens:

From estrogen:
- nausea
- breast enlargement and tenderness
- uterine bleeding, sometimes irregular, usually diminishing with time
- headache
- fluid retention

From progestogens:
- depression
- mood changes

Unfortunately, women who use estrogen after menopause and women who use oral contraceptives both have an increased risk of serious gallbladder disease.[30, 31, 32]

Some women take estrogen as a vaginal cream or skin patch. When estrogen is absorbed in this way, it largely bypasses the liver, and both liver and gallbladder problems are usually avoided.

Estrogen Therapy Increases Your Risk of Having a Hysterectomy

Women who take estrogen alone are eight times more likely to experience vaginal bleeding episodes than are women who go through natural menopause and choose

Reasons Not to Use Hormone Therapy

Women who are considering taking hormone replacement therapy for severe menopausal symptoms or as a means to prevent osteoporosis should consider avoiding it if they have any of the following conditions:

1. past or present thromboembolic events such as stroke, thrombophlebitis, pulmonary embolus, heart attack
2. breast cancer, history of advanced endometrial cancer, any other estrogen-stimulated cancer
3. impairment of liver function
4. unexplained vaginal bleeding
5. pregnancy or chance of pregnancy
6. gallbladder disease
7. uterine fibroids that become or remain symptomatic on hormones
8. hypertension
9. migraines that worsen on hormones

not to take any hormones. Hysterectomy — sometimes used to control bleeding—is six times more likely in women who use estrogen alone.[33] Women who take estrogen plus a progestogen have no increased risk of hysterectomy.[34] Without further research and more data on why women take estrogens, it is difficult to interpret the meaning of this association.

Hormone Therapy Increases Your Risk of Blood Clots

Both estrogen and estrogen plus a progestogen seem to be associated with blood clots. Several studies have found a higher incidence of venous thromboembolism (blood clots in veins that can travel to the lung and cause pulmonary emboli).[35, 36, 37, 38] These events are serious, even fatal, but uncommon. The relationship between ERT/HRT and stroke is less clear. Most studies show no influence on the incidence of stroke.[39, 40, 41]

Hormone Therapy May Increase Your Risk of Getting Asthma

Two reports have shown a relationship between ERT/HRT use and asthma. In the Nurses Health Study, women who choose to use either estrogen alone or estrogen plus a progestogen have about a 50 percent higher risk of developing asthma.[42] Long-term use seems to increase the risk a little bit more. In a small

> Both estrogen and estrogen plus a progestogen seem to be associated with blood clots.

study, fifteen women with asthma were tested before and during a month-long trial of estrogen.[43] These women were less able to take a deep breath while on ERT, although it didn't affect the way they felt during the short duration of the study. This issue needs further examination to determine whether or not increased asthma risk is a real effect of ERT/HRT.

Hormone Therapy May Increase Your Risk of Getting Lupus

Lupus is an unusual disease in which our immune defenses turn against our own bodies. It is much more common among women than men and seems in some way associated with hormones. Researchers from the Nurses Health Study looked at the experience of women who chose to use ERT or HRT and found they have higher rates of lupus.[44] A more recent study in Great Britain found that two or more years of ERT significantly increased the likelihood of developing lupus.[45] Further research, including consideration of the reasons why these women took the hormones, is needed to explore the contributing factors to this association.

CHAPTER FIVE

Designer Estrogens
How Do We Calculate the Odds?

The potential benefit is real, but so far it is unfulfilled.

Now that millions of baby boomers are at midlife, they are the focus of a great deal of product marketing related to aging. That includes pharmaceuticals. With so many women reluctant to use medication because of concerns about side effects and risks, how will the drug companies continue to talk us out of our dollars?

For menopausal women, the pharmaceutical industry's answer is to develop high-benefit, low-risk compounds that offer all the benefits of estrogen without the risks. Many companies are now devoting large portions of their research budgets to do just that.

One such category of drugs that some researchers and companies believe will achieve this goal is the SERMs (selective estrogen receptor modulators). Often referred to as "designer estrogens," SERMs have different effects on estrogen receptors at different sites. In some parts of the body, they have anti-estrogenic effects, while in others, they are estrogenic.

Tamoxifen

The best-known designer estrogen is tamoxifen, an anti-estrogen used to treat breast cancer and prevent its recurrence. While tamoxifen has anti-estrogenic effects in the breast, it has estrogenic effects on bone and to some extent on cholesterol. It maintains bone density in postmenopausal women, and it lowers artery-clogging LDL cholesterol, though it does not increase beneficial HDL as estrogen does.

On the negative side, tamoxifen's estrogenic effects increase the risk of serious blood clots and stimulate cell growth in the endometrium, increasing the odds of endometrial cancer. Unlike estrogen, it increases hot flashes.

Often referred to as "designer estrogens," SERMs have different effects on estrogen receptors at different sites. In some parts of the body, they have anti-estrogenic effects, while in others, they are estrogenic.

In 1998, the FDA approved tamoxifen for use by women at high risk for breast cancer as a way to reduce their risk of getting the disease. The FDA based its approval primarily on a study that followed women for approximately four years and showed a 49 percent reduced risk of invasive breast cancer.[1] In the same study, however, women taking tamoxifen had over two and a half times more endometrial cancer, three times more pulmonary emboli, and one and half times more strokes and deep venous thromboses than women taking the placebo.

For young women at extremely high risk of getting breast cancer, tamoxifen lives up to the theoretical promise of SERMs by reducing the risk of cancer more than it increases the risk of other serious health problems. Blood clots, stroke, and endometrial cancer are all rare in women under age fifty, and no unexpected cases appeared in this study. In most older women with no risk factors other than age, however, the negative effects of taking the drug outweighed the benefits. Blood clots and endometrial cancer are more common in older women, and the increased numbers of women with these problems outweigh the number of breast cancers delayed in all but a very small group of older women at extremely high risk.[2]

> For young women at extremely high risk of getting breast cancer, tamoxifen lives up to the theoretical promise of SERMs by reducing the risk of cancer more than it increases the risk of other serious health problems.

Even though tamoxifen is far from perfect, it indicates the potential for SERMs.

Raloxifene

Another SERM, raloxifene, produced by Eli Lilly under the brand name Evista, is widely promoted to health care providers and women as a way to prevent bone fractures. In early ads to consumers that didn't even name the drug, Lilly created the impression that it offered the benefits of estrogen (increased bone density and improved blood lipid profile) without the risks of endometrial or breast cancer. This is a message with obvious appeal both to consumers and practitioners, but is it true?

From a two-year study of 601 early postmenopausal women comparing raloxifene to placebo, researchers concluded that in the raloxifene group, bone mineral density increased, while artery-clogging LDL cholesterol and total cholesterol decreased, and there was no stimulation of the endometrium that could lead to endometrial cancer. No changes occurred in artery-scrubbing HDL cholesterol or destructive triglyceride levels either—the drug provided neither the beneficial increase in HDL nor the harmful increase in triglycerides that estrogen does. Compared with a placebo, there was no significant difference in hot flashes or vaginal bleeding, though the authors of the study did report that in other unpublished trials, women experienced higher levels of hot flashes.[3]

The FDA approved raloxifene for prevention of osteoporosis in postmenopausal women. While increased bone density does not necessarily lead to decreased fracture risk, recent research on raloxifene has found a dose-related reduction in vertebral fracture detected by X-ray, but not in other fractures.[4] In another study of raloxifene, a 60 mg/day dose decreased vertebral fractures by 30 percent, while a 120 mg/day dose decreased them by 50 percent.[5]

In humans, no study of raloxifene has shown an increase in breast cancer. In fact, the first studies appear to show a decrease.

There are some negative side effects to raloxifene described in Eli Lilly's patient information packet. Raloxifene increases the risk of blood clots, and the company advises anyone with a history of blood clots not to take it. There is also a warning to stop taking raloxifene at least three days before "you plan on being immobile for a long time" because of the increased risk of blood clots. This warning may be challenging to act on since breaking one's hip and many other things that cause immobility are not planned events.

The full potential benefits of raloxifene may not yet be known. Some studies suggest it may *reduce* the risk of breast cancer. It inhibits production of human breast cancer cells *in vitro* and the development of certain mammary tumors in rats.[6]

At a December 1998 breast cancer symposium, V.C. Jordan, a researcher at Northwestern University, reported on a meta-analysis of raloxifene trials on osteoporosis prevention involving 10,575 postmenopausal women. According to his report, while there were no differences in breast cancer rates in the first six months of treatment, after six months, benefits appeared. Breast cancer rates fell significantly with raloxifene (from 3.8 per 1,000 patient-years in the placebo group to 1.7) after a median follow-up of forty months.[7] Jordan leads the STAR (Study of Tamoxifen and Raloxifene) Trial that is comparing tamoxifen and raloxifene in postmenopausal women who are at risk for breast cancer.

It is important to note that the data on raloxifene's effect on breast cancer is still too short-term to support reliable conclusions about its long-term safety or benefit. The experience to date with tamoxifen shows why: When used as treatment for women with breast

STAR: A Trial of New Estrogens

Raloxifene is being studied in a large trial financed solely by the federal government. The trial is called STAR (Study of Tamoxifen and Raloxifene).

Researchers began recruiting women for the trial in 1999 and hope that 16,000 women in all will volunteer. The trial evaluates the effects of these two drugs on two groups of postmenopausal women who so far are healthy but are at higher-than-average risk of breast cancer. One group takes tamoxifen (Nolvadex); the other takes raloxifene (Evista). There is no placebo group. Women taking part in STAR agree to take their pills (they look exactly alike) for five years, the amount of time researchers calculate will reveal any difference in the rate of breast cancer between the two groups.

This trial, in its current design, is opposed by the National Women's Health Network, as well as by two cancer activist groups, Breast Cancer Action and the National Breast Cancer Coalition.

These groups object to the basic assumption of the STAR trial that tamoxifen is already proven to be useful to

cancer, tamoxifen has beneficial effects in preventing recurrence of breast cancer at two years and at five years, but its effect reverses by ten years.

This means that women who have had breast cancer and are taking tamoxifen to prevent recurrence may have a higher rate of recurrence if they take tamoxifen for ten years than if they take it for five years. While seemingly counterintuitive, this demonstrates why consumers and healthy women and that the only question to answer now is whether raloxifene is better. The activists insist that tamoxifen has *not* been proven useful to healthy women and that those who enroll in the study are being misled. They contend the women are exchanging their hope of not getting breast cancer for an increased risk of endometrial cancer (if they have a uterus), stroke, and pulmonary embolism.

On the other hand, many women's health advocates believe that women can't know tamoxifen's potential usefulness to them unless researchers study what happens after women take it for five years. Many crucial questions about tamoxifen remain unanswered:

- Does tamoxifen save lives?
- Do the breast cancer cases prevented during the five years women are on tamoxifen appear soon after they stop taking the drug?
- As more time elapses, will healthy women experience even more harmful effects than those seen during the study?

practitioners should use caution and avoid relying on short-term trials to assess long-term benefits or risks. Good news in the short run may become no news—or bad news—in the long run.

We believe it's premature to recommend raloxifene for fracture prevention, despite promising early results and FDA approval. Its beneficial effects on lipid profile do not yet show up as a reduction in heart attacks, for example, yet there has been a clear and demonstrated increase in life-threatening blood clots in the lungs and elsewhere.

Many researchers agree that long-term, large, randomized studies are needed before any benefits can be confirmed, and we agree.[8, 9] Our position is that studies lasting at least ten years are needed to show whether or not raloxifene is truly "safe" for prevention of osteoporosis and that the evidence is insufficient to promote raloxifene as a drug that prevents heart disease or breast cancer.

> We believe it's premature to recommend raloxifene for fracture prevention, despite promising early results and FDA approval.

Unfortunately, before raloxifene's safety and benefits have been thoroughly researched, direct-to-consumer advertising is already promoting it as "safer" than estrogen.

In the meantime, other drug companies are developing other SERMs, and it is clear that this will be a major focus of new research. In the coming years, as each new SERM comes onto the market with the accompanying hype of multimillion dollar advertising campaigns, consumers will need to recognize the limitations of short-term studies in demonstrating both the benefits and risks of these drugs.

PART TWO

What Remedies Relieve Perimenopausal and Menopausal Symptoms?

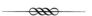

CHAPTER SIX

Hormone Therapy for Relief of Menopausal Symptoms

When other remedies don't work, some women choose to take small amounts of HRT for short periods of time.

Drop into almost any women's menopausal support group, and the problem you're most likely to hear about is hot flashes.

"I'm a mess—hot flashes wake me up every couple of hours and then I can't get back to sleep. I never get more than four hours sleep a night."

"Sex is a bust—hot flashes drove my husband out of bed and onto the living room couch."

"I'm pissed. Hot flashes have me so irritable that I feel like I'm going to kick the next person I see."

Although hot flashes are serious business, they aren't the only symptoms that make menopausal and perimenopausal women uncomfortable. Heavy bleeding, vaginal dryness, and itching and thinning of the vaginal wall also contribute their share of grief and make life more unpredictable than we'd like.[1]

> For many women, the decision of how to take estrogen requires nearly as much thought as the decision whether to take it at all.

Most of these discomforts are transient, lasting only until our bodies adjust from the premenopausal to postmenopausal state. Few bother us significantly, and all tend to improve with time. However, some women who experience intense distress during menopause understandably look for remedies. Here's how estrogen and hormone replacement therapy can help.

Estrogen for Hot Flashes and Vaginal Dryness

First of all, estrogen relieves hot flashes and vaginal dryness in most women and is approved by the FDA for these conditions. It has many forms, with the pill, the patch, and vaginal cream all in general use in the United States. The most common types are conjugated estrogens (a mixture of estrogens) and micronized estradiol (a synthetically produced form of estrogen that is chemically identical to the estrogen produced by our ovaries). Dosages vary.

For many women, the decision of how to take estrogen requires nearly as much thought as the decision whether to take it at all.

To minimize your risk of problems (see page 45 in chapter 4, "The Risks of Hormone Replacement Therapy"), it's important to find the lowest dose that gives you relief. Lower dose forms are equally effective in relieving hot flashes and improving vaginal atrophy.[2] If you begin taking a standard dose of HRT and find that you are getting relief, you might ask your physician for a lower dose to see if that works as well.

> Any woman who's been advised not to use estrogen should consult a health care provider before using the cream or the patch.

Topical Vaginal Estrogen Relieves Dryness

While clinicians frequently prescribe pills and patches for hot flashes, they may recommend pills, vaginal estrogen cream, or rings for treatment of vaginal dryness, itching, and thinning of the vaginal walls. These problems all respond to topical vaginal estrogen.

Estrogen in the topical creams and rings goes directly and quickly into the bloodstream, affecting the whole body, not just the vagina.[3] However, vaginal estrogen products produce lower blood levels than the pill form. Any woman who's been advised not to use estrogen

If You're Considering Hormone Therapy

Women who are on estrogen alone or on combined estrogen and progestogens should plan to visit their clinicians regularly. If, after careful consideration, these women decide they want to stop taking hormones, they should lower the dosage gradually over a few months to avoid a sudden drop in hormone levels and possible resumption of hot flashes.

Here is a list of questions to ask before beginning hormone therapy.

1. Why is the doctor prescribing it for me? Am I at risk for osteoporosis? Do I have severe discomfort? Have I tried natural ways of coping with my menopause?
2. What kinds of tests and questions should be included in the medical evaluation prior to my use of hormone therapy?
3. What are the contraindications to this regimen? Do I have any of these contraindications?
4. What is the dosage, and how long will the treatment last? Is the prescribed dosage as low as possible? If I am taking estrogen for a surgically induced menopause, will the dosage be decreased to mimic natural menopause as I grow older?
5. If I take hormone therapy, what additional medical tests do I need, and how often does my clinician need to monitor the hormones' effects on me? If I am on hormones, how will it affect my mammograms?
6. What is the cost for follow-up care?
7. What can I do, myself, to avoid use of hormone therapy? What are my alternatives?

should consult a health care provider before using the cream or the patch.

Some women being treated for cancer choose to use a minimal dose of estrogen cream to relieve vaginal dryness. Because estrogen affects the growth of many cancers, most doctors exercise extreme caution in prescribing it for a woman undergoing cancer treatment.

A Gradual Approach

Making a decision for or against hormone use for menopausal complaints depends on your individual situation. Many women choose to try alternative remedies first and only move on to drugs if other approaches don't work or are not available to them. These women use hormones to control the transition from pre- to post-menopause by taking gradually reduced amounts for as short a time as possible.

Hot flashes may recur after cessation of hormone therapy, especially if a woman stops taking the drugs suddenly.

Yet even short-term use of ERT and HRT has risks. A letter to participants in the Women's Health Initiative (WHI) in 2001 warned that those receiving either ERT or HRT were at increased risk for heart attacks and blood clots or strokes during the first three years of use, compared with women receiving a placebo. The study coordinator sent the letter to all of the women participating in the clinical trial because the results were unexpected and were not included in the consent form given to the women when they enrolled. The data are not sufficient to stop the study or to conclude definitively that estrogen causes these problems, but they are significant enough that WHI felt an ethical obligation to inform participants. One can't draw conclusions about this possible risk until the study is completed, but these disturbing preliminary results undercut the hope that short-term use of estrogen can be risk-free.

Hot flashes may recur after cessation of hormone therapy, especially if a woman stops taking the drugs suddenly.

ERT and HRT seem to help some women who experience heavy bleeding in the years leading up to and during menopause.

Some women experience anxiety, moodiness, and/or irritability during menopause, and HRT seems not to have an impact on that either. This is discussed in greater detail in chapter 12 ("Will Hormone Therapy Preserve Mind, Mood, and Memory?").

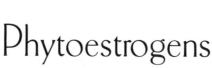

CHAPTER SEVEN

Phytoestrogens
Help for Some

Will phytoestrogens relieve your symptoms? Can they prevent disease?

When writer Ellen Watts got an upper respiratory infection just before her forty-ninth birthday, she had a fever, congestion, and a cough. She bounced back within a few days, except that every couple of nights the "fever" seemed to return, waking her up and making sleep impossible.

A month later, desperate for sleep and concerned that she was brewing a secondary infection, Ellen saw her doctor, who prescribed some antibiotics. "They didn't seem to help," she says now. When she skipped her period six months later, she finally realized the recurring "fever" was a series of hot flashes, plain and simple.

Once Ellen knew she was dealing with menopause, she started looking for a way to stop the flashes. A dietician friend who knew how much Ellen loved an early morning latte suggested that she start making her latte with soymilk. That way Ellen would get a small slug of

Do You Speak Soy?

For those who have not yet explored the world of soy, here's a translation of the terms used on the labels of various soy products:

- **Green soybeans.** Fresh soybeans, usually eaten boiled (also called edamame).

- **Miso.** Fermented bean paste, used as a base for Japanese soups and sauces.

- **Soy grits, soy flour, soy powder.** Different particle sizes of soybeans (usually made from defatted soybean flakes).

- **Soymilk.** A milk substitute made from cooked soybeans. American varieties may contain various flavorings.

- **Soy protein concentrate.** Usually contains 65 percent protein. Prepared from defatted soybeans and used in many commercially prepared soy products.

phytoestrogens—estrogens that occur in soybeans and other plants—to help counteract the fluctuations of her own estrogen that were causing the hot flashes.

From then on, every morning Ellen heated six ounces of soymilk in the microwave, added a tablespoon of freeze-dried coffee and a tablespoon of Hershey's milk chocolate syrup. "It wasn't Starbucks," admits Ellen, "but it was darned good." The strategy worked. The phytoestrogens kept her "fever" down so she slept through the night.

- **Soy protein isolate.** A 90 percent protein product prepared from defatted soybeans. Used in infant formulas as well as many commercially prepared soy products.
- **Tempeh.** A fermented, firm tofu product usually packaged in blocks.
- **Textured soy protein.** May be made from isolates, concentrates, soy grits or soy flour. Often processed to resemble different sorts of meat.
- **Tofu.** This is your basic bean curd. Made by adding a coagulant to the liquid squeezed from cooked soybeans, it's a bland and versatile Asian food that comes in many forms. Usually sold in blocks and labeled as to texture, ranging from "silken" (very soft, used in shakes and puddings) to soft, firm, and extra firm. Softer types are usually used in soups and the firmer type in stir-fries and casseroles. There are many varieties of pressed, dried, and fermented tofu.

Grains, Beans, and Seeds

Phytoestrogens are much weaker estrogens than the ones we make in our own bodies, having only about 1/200th the strength of our own. However, a diet rich in these substances is frequently all it takes to ride comfortably through menopause.

There are two main kinds of phytoestrogens: lignans and isoflavones. Incidentally, when we talk about precursors here and elsewhere, we mean the substances

> ## Legumes Cut Endometrial
> ## Cancer Risk in Half
>
> Phytoestrogens, unlike pharmaceutical estrogens, do
> not appear to increase endometrial cancer rates. A case-
> control, observational study compared various dietary
> factors in 332 endometrial cancer patients in Hawaii and
> 511 age- and ethnicity-matched controls.[1] The subjects
> were Japanese, Caucasian, Chinese, Filipino, and native
> Hawaiians. High consumption of soy and other legumes
> was associated with cutting in half the risk of developing
> endometrial cancer. High fiber and low-fat diets also cor-
> related with reduced risk.

from which other substances are formed. Lignan precursors are found in whole grains, seeds, fruits, and vegetables—especially flaxseed, rye, millet, and legumes.
Isoflavone precursors are found in soybeans, chickpeas,
and other legumes.[2,3] Bacteria in our intestines convert
plant lignans to mammalian lignans (enterolactone and
enterodiol) and convert isoflavone precursors to active
isoflavones (genistein, daidzein, and equol).

Other phytoestrogens occur in some medicinal herbs,
but these are different from the phytoestrogens in food
plants, and, in terms of safety, we should treat them differently (see chapter 8, "Herbs," and chapter 16, "Alternatives to Hormone Replacement Therapy").

In Asia, consumption of such legumes as soybeans,
other beans, lentils, and peas provides 25 to 45 mg of

total isoflavones a day, compared with Western countries where average consumption is less than 5 mg a day. Soybeans, mainly in the form of fresh, dried, pressed, or fermented tofu, are a common food in China, Japan, Korea, and other Asian countries. In Japan, where soy consumption is very high, people consume up to 200 mg of isoflavones daily.[4]

Phytoestrogens Control Hot Flashes

Asian women complain less of hot flashes than do Western women, and it may be that eating soy products has some effects similar to hormone replacement therapy.[5] Most but not all studies have shown that supplementing one's diet with phytoestrogens can help hot flashes and vaginal dryness.

A randomized, double-blind, placebo-controlled study of 104 postmenopausal women found that 60 grams of isolated soy protein taken for twelve weeks reduced hot flashes by 45 percent. This compared with a 30 percent reduction in the placebo group treated with 60 grams a day of the milk protein casein,[6] a statistically significant difference. The differences between the two groups began appearing at

> In Asia, consumption of such legumes as soybeans, other beans, lentils, and peas provides 25 to 45 mg of total isoflavones a day, compared with Western countries where average consumption is less than 5 mg a day.

three weeks. Adverse effects, mainly in the form of gas-trointestinal complaints, were similar in the two groups.

A second study, this one by Brzezinski of 145 Israeli women with menopausal symptoms, found that the seventy-eight women assigned to a phytoestrogen-rich diet had fewer hot flashes and less vaginal dryness than thirty-six women in the control group who did not change their diet. The study lasted twelve weeks. Women in the treatment group substituted phytoestrogen-rich foods, including tofu, soy drink, miso, and flaxseed, for approximately one-fourth of their daily caloric intake.[7]

Murkies's study of fifty-eight women compared intake of 45 grams of soy flour daily against 45 grams of wheat flour for twelve weeks. The soy group had significantly fewer hot flashes.[8]

Finally, Dalais's double-blind, randomized, placebo-controlled, crossover trial studied fifty-two post-menopausal women (forty-four of whom completed the study) ages forty-five to sixty-five. The women had more than fourteen hot flashes a week. They tested 45 grams per day (in the form of bread) of soy grits baked in bread (containing 53 mg per day of isoflavones), linseed (as flaxseed), or wheat meal (as a placebo) for twelve weeks.[9] Researchers looked at hot flash frequency, bone mineral content (BMC), bone mineral density (BMD), and vaginal maturation index (VMI), which is a measure of estrogenic effect. (Estrogen makes postmenopausal vaginal cells look more like premenopausal vaginal cells, reflected by a higher VMI. If vaginal thinning makes sex uncomfortable, a higher VMI may help, but a direct correlation has not been shown.)

Compared with baseline, soy did not change the number of hot flashes, but it did increase the VMI by 103 percent and increased bone mineral density by 5.2 percent. Linseed decreased hot flashes 41 percent ($p<0.009$) but had no effect on VMI, bone mineral density, or bone mineral content. Wheat decreased hot flashes 51 percent ($p<0.001$); there was no change in the vaginal maturation index, BMD, or BMC. (For explanation of p values, shown in parentheses, see appendix A.)

Not every trial showed phytoestrogen benefits. A double-blind, placebo-controlled, crossover trial of fifty-one perimenopausal women ages forty-five to fifty-five who were having more than one hot flash a day tested the effect of 20 grams of soy protein (with 34 mg phytoestrogens) taken once daily or divided into two doses. Each phase lasted six weeks. Compared with the placebo phase, during which women received 20 grams of complex carbohydrate without phytoestrogens, there was no difference in hot flash frequency among the different phases. However, hot flash severity was significantly lower during the split-dose soy phase ($p<0.001$).

As an added benefit, during the soy phases, total cholesterol and LDL cholesterol decreased ($p<0.01$). Diastolic blood pressure was also significantly lowered ($p<0.01$) during the split-dose phase.[10]

Phytoestrogens and Vaginal Health

Four studies have looked at whether supplementing the diet with phytoestrogens resulted in estrogenic changes

Food or Supplements?

Soy foods have been a staple in Asian cuisine for thousands of years and can be presumed safe, at least for those raised on it. There is some interesting evidence that phytoestrogen consumption during puberty, when breasts develop, could be the most critical period for its intake. Beans are safe; the recent availability of purified isoflavone, mixed-phytoestrogen, or nonfood phytoestrogen pills like red clover, however, is worrisome. There is no long-term safety data available for these food-free phytoestrogens, and we discourage their use.

in vaginal cells, which may relieve the discomfort that some women experience at menopause. Two studies were positive and two were negative.

A study of twenty-five women tested 45 grams of soy flour daily and found significant estrogenic changes.[11] Of the studies discussed previously, the Brzezinski study also found improvements in vaginal cells. The Dalais study found a benefit for soy but not flax. The Murkies study did not find significant changes in vaginal cells.

In another study, ninety-one women took textured vegetable protein and dried soybeans amounting to a daily intake of 165 mg of isoflavones. The results did not show a significant difference between the soy group compared with the controls.[12] This study apparently used an unusual method of collecting vaginal cells that may have undercounted estrogenized cells.

Do Phytoestrogens Prevent Breast Cancer?

Even though soybeans and other phytoestrogens are being touted as breast cancer preventatives, the evidence is not very clear. Women should be wary of phytoestrogen supplements proliferating on drugstore shelves, because those supplements may have very different effects than adding tofu to meals.

Experimental data supports the view that phytoestrogens, because they are natural selective estrogen modulators (SERMs), may have a protective effect against breast cancer. In laboratory tests, the phytoestrogen genistein seems to suppress the growth of many types of cancer cells.[13]

Studies of breast cancer in animals, however, show mixed results.[14] Several epidemiological studies show a protective effect of soy consumption on breast cancer risk, but the results are not entirely consistent. Studies of different human populations show that groups that consume a lot of phytoestrogens have a lower rate of breast cancer, but this protective effect may be strongest in premenopausal women. For example:

> Women should be wary of phytoestrogen supplements proliferating on drugstore shelves, because they may have very different effects than adding tofu to meals.

- A case-control study that compared food choices of 200 Chinese women in Singapore who had breast cancer with 420 matched controls found that soy product intake had a protective effect in

premenopausal women but no effect on postmenopausal women.[15]

- Another case-control study of premenopausal and
  postmenopausal women in China did not find a
  protective effect in either group.[16]

- A recent case-control study of 288 premenopausal
  and postmenopausal women found that those with
  breast cancer consumed fewer phytoestrogens
  (measured by the amount excreted in their urine)
  than women without breast cancer.[17]

- In a study of postmenopausal women, phytoestrogen
  supplementation markedly increased sex-hormone-
  binding globulin (SHBG). High levels of SHBG are
  associated with lower breast cancer risk.[18]

Finally, one rather peculiar epidemiological study
found a protective effect of miso (fermented soy paste) on
breast cancer in a Japanese population living in Hawaii.[19]
The major problem with that study is that it calculated
the dietary intake of *husbands* as a surrogate for their
spouses. It is usually true that couples who eat together
have similar diets. However, in a number of these cases,
the spouse was already dead and thus unavailable as a dinner companion!

The Effect of Phytoestrogens on Breast Cancer Survivors

The claim by some that consuming foods containing
phytoestrogens is dangerous is clearly absurd. Asian
women have consumed such food for thousands of years

and have a lower risk of breast cancer than Western women of all ages.

What is not clear is whether the estrogenic properties of soybeans can cause breast cancer to grow. What's more, the effect of phytoestrogens may be different in premenopausal and postmenopausal women because of different "background" estrogen levels. There is

> We believe that supplementing your diet with beans, whole grains, and flaxseed and other foods containing phytoestrogens is safe.

some interesting evidence that phytoestrogen consumption during puberty, when breasts develop, could be the most critical period.

In any case, here's what we know so far: In a laboratory study of cultured breast cancer cells, both estradiol and a phytoestrogen stimulated cell growth. When they were added together, however, little to no growth stimulation occurred. In a mouse model with a damaged immune system, phytoestrogen implants caused estrogen-receptor-positive (but not estrogen-receptor-negative) breast cancer implants to grow.[20] It's not clear that this is a good model for predicting results in humans, but it is what we have.

Although few data are available, we believe that supplementing your diet with beans, whole grains, and flaxseed and other foods containing phytoestrogens is safe. We see no need for postmenopausal women with breast cancer to actively avoid phytoestrogens. After all, they are an important part of the diet in many countries with low breast cancer rates and are found in many foods with high nutritive value. We also feel, however, that phytoestrogen pills should be avoided.

Should breast cancer patients who are being treated with the hormonal drug tamoxifen take phytoestrogens as a supplement? These two substances have similar effects in terms of having some estrogenic and some antiestrogenic properties. There are no human studies on whether combining the use of phytoestrogens and tamoxifen has a beneficial or deleterious effect. What's more, isoflavone supplementation does not appear to help hot flashes in breast cancer survivors.

In a randomized, double-blind, placebo-controlled crossover trial, 177 women who had a history of breast cancer and at least fourteen hot flashes per week (156 of the women were currently using tamoxifen) were treated with three soy tablets daily. Each 600 mg tablet contained 50 mg of soy isoflavones. Total intake of isoflavones was thus 150 mg per day. One hundred forty-nine women completed the study. The trial was nine weeks long. The first week was to establish a baseline, then women received four weeks of either the treatment or the placebo. After that, the subjects crossed over to the other substance.[21]

Percentages of patients reporting reductions in hot flashes were similar between the two groups. The percentage of patients reporting a 50 percent reduction in hot flash frequency was significantly higher in the group taking the placebo (36 percent) than in the group receiving soy (24 percent). Patients did not prefer soy to the placebo. There were no significant differences between the two groups regarding gastrointestinal symptoms.

This study found no benefit using isoflavone pills for hot flashes in breast cancer survivors, most of whom were taking tamoxifen. For women with breast cancer, we believe that a case can be made either for supplementing or avoiding supplemental phytoestrogens and that the most prudent decision may be to do neither.

Soy Is a Joy to Your Heart

Soybeans may help prevent cardiovascular disease. An FDA ruling in the year 2000 determined that foods containing 6.25 grams or more of soy protein can claim that, as part of a diet low in saturated fat and cholesterol, soy protein may reduce the risk of coronary heart disease.

A meta-analysis of thirty-eight controlled clinical trials found that eating a lot of soy protein helped reduce overall cholesterol (9.3 percent less than controls), LDL cholesterol (12.9 percent), and triglycerides (10.5 percent). HDL cholesterol was unaffected.[22]

In animals, cardiovascular risk factors seem to diminish with use of phytoestrogens. One study comparing Premarin with phytoestrogens randomized 189 macaque monkeys with surgically induced menopause into three groups.[23] All were fed a fatty diet. One group ate a soy diet with 1.7 mg/kg isoflavones, the second group ate an isoflavone-free soy diet, and the third group ate a soy-free diet and received estrogen in a dose equivalent to conjugated estrogens at 0.625 mg a day.

The soy diet with isoflavones had about the same effect on blood lipids as the conjugated estrogens, although soy was superior to conjugated estrogens in increasing apolipoprotein A-1, which is associated with HDL, the "good" cholesterol. It did not cause an increase in triglycerides, a common side effect of conjugated estrogens.

The investigators also found a beneficial effect equivalent to that of conjugated estrogens from the soy diet on coronary artery reactivity, which is the tendency for arteries to go into spasm, a known risk factor for heart attack. In a study of twenty-two atherosclerotic rhesus monkeys, the investigators fed all monkeys a soy-based diet with half of the monkeys receiving isoflavone-free soy and the others receiving soy with isoflavones.

The result? The arteries of females in the isoflavone group had a better response than the isoflavone-free group to a drug that usually causes constriction.

Osteoporosis: The Jury's Still Out

Epidemiologically, bone density is lowest in Asian women and highest in African American women, with white women in the middle. That should mean that Asian women are prone to fractures, but it doesn't.

Instead, hip fracture rates are lower in Asians than in whites,[24] even though they have thinner bones and their calcium intake is far lower than Western women.

Compared with white women, Asian women have a 40 to 50 percent lower risk of hip fracture, and African Americans a 50 to 60 percent lower risk.[25] The reasons for these differences are unknown, although body mass, differences in hip axis length, and bone quality may all play a role. (It is possible that high soy intake contributes to better bone quality in Asians compared with whites, but this is entirely speculative: There are many differences between these two groups.) It

> It bears noting that bone density measurements are only one indicator of fragility: Bone quality may matter as much as bone quantity.

bears noting that bone density measurements are only one indicator of fragility (see chapter 10, "Hormone Therapy and Osteoporosis"). Bone quality may matter as much as bone quantity.[26]

Clinical Trials

In a double-blind study of postmenopausal women ages forty-nine to seventy-three with high cholesterol,[27] the sixty-six participants were randomly assigned to 40 grams of protein a day from one of three sources: nonfat dried milk and casein, soy protein with medium isoflavone content (equivalent to 55.6 mg isoflavones daily), or isolated soy protein with high isoflavone content (equivalent to 90 mg isoflavones daily) for six months. All the women also followed a low-fat, low-cholesterol diet.

No differences were seen among the three groups in bone density studies of the hip and total body, but subjects receiving the high isoflavone preparation experienced a significant increase in lumbar bone density and mineral content (2 percent), compared with the milk protein group.

Another randomized, double-blind study assigned sixty-nine women to take soy, isoflavone-free soy, or whey protein (as a control) for twenty-four weeks.[28] Compared with baseline, only the control group had a significant decrease in BMD and BMC. Soy with intact isoflavones appeared to be particularly beneficial.

Animal Studies

In rats, both soybean intake and genistein (the major isoflavone in beans) have positive effects on bone density.[29, 30, 31] Apparently, genistein stimulates bone growth. It is a different mechanism from estrogen, which inhibits bone breakdown.[32]

Another study in which rats were injected with genistein found similar results: less bone loss in the genistein-treated group and a higher rate of bone formation without any effect on bone resorption.[33]

Genistein may have different results at different doses and may be more effective when one takes less rather than more. One study performed a total assault on bone mineral stores by feeding a low-calcium diet to four groups of lactating rats whose ovaries were surgically removed. Generally, rats so treated will lose more than 50 percent of bone mineral mass in two weeks. The groups received one of three different doses of genistein (0.5 mg, 1.6 mg, and 5.0 mg daily) or conjugated estrogen.[34] The rats receiving low-dose genistein had the heaviest and most dense bones of all the rats studied. In other words, genistein at a low dose was more effective at preserving bone than at a higher dose.

While most rat studies show beneficial effects of soy or genistein on bone, a study of primates did not.[35] This coincides with other animal studies showing inconsistent results about the preservation of bone density. One consistent finding is that soy, unlike estrogen, does not reduce oophorectomy-induced bone turnover. Soy's beneficial effect appears to be in stimulating bone formation rather than reducing bone resorption.

Although we lack definitive evidence that dietary soy or isoflavone supplementation benefits bone, one reasonable study on humans shows a modest effect from high-isoflavone soy supplementation on spinal (not hip) bone.[36] In any case, there is enough intriguing evidence about animals to warrant further clinical research into soy's activity in humans. We also need long-term human studies comparing the effect of HRT or bisphosphonates with soy supplementation on fracture incidence to determine whether phytoestrogens protect bone.

> Soy's beneficial effect appears to be in stimulating bone formation rather than reducing bone resorption.

If You Want to Supplement with Phytoestrogens

You can significantly increase your intake of lignans by eating more whole grains—especially rye—and by sprinkling a tablespoon of freshly ground flaxseed over your cereal and salad every day.

Soybeans, chickpeas (also called garbanzo beans), lima beans, other beans, and peas are excellent sources of isoflavones. And although soybeans are a rich source of phytoestrogens, other legumes are even better sources of genistein and daidzein.[37, 38] Anasazi, brown, black, navy, pinto, and turtle beans contain almost similar amounts of genistein as soybeans, with much less fat.[39]

Most beans contain 1 percent fat, compared with 18 to 20 percent fat in soy. This breaks down to 15 percent saturated fat, 23 percent monounsaturated fats, and 58 percent polyunsaturated fatty acids.[40]

How much of these phytoestrogens do you need? No one really knows, although we can get a clue by looking at the amounts used by researchers in the studies mentioned earlier. In Asia, consumption of legumes provides 25 to 200 mg of total isoflavones a day.[41]

If you're trying to increase the isoflavones in your diet, keep in mind that not all soy products are equal in isoflavone content. Soy oil and soy sauce contain inconsequential amounts of isoflavones. Fermented soy products often have fewer isoflavones than unfermented products, but fermentation appears to increase how well they are absorbed. To see the isoflavone content of foods, take a look at the table in the box titled "Where to Find Phytoestrogens."

One question people frequently ask is whether low-fat soy products retain isoflavones. Actually, isoflavones are not very fat soluble, which is why soy oil is almost devoid of isoflavones. Therefore, removing the fat does not remove a lot of isoflavones. What can make a difference

Where to Find Phytoestrogens

It's difficult for most of us to figure out which plant food is likely to have the concentration of phytoestrogens we want. The table below may give you a start. It lists the levels of two important phytoestrogens found in the seeds of several common plants.

Seed	Genistein (ppm)	Daidzein (ppm)	Genistein per 4-oz serving	Daidzein per 4-oz serving
Yellow split pea	45.8	0.4	5.2 mg	0.05 mg
Black turtle beans	45.1	0.4	5.125 mg	0.05 mg
Baby lima beans	40.1	0.4	4.56 mg	0.05 mg
Large lima beans	34.4	0.3	3.91 mg	0.03 mg
Anasazi beans	29.8	6.5	3.39 mg	0.74 mg
Red kidney beans	29.3	2.7	3.33 mg	0.31 mg
Red lentils	25.0	5.2	2.84 mg	0.59 mg
Soybeans	24.1	37.6	2.74 mg	4.3 mg
Black-eyed peas	23.3	0.3	2.65 mg	0.03 mg
Pinto beans	22.3	23.2	2.53 mg	2.64 mg
Mung beans	21.8	0.3	2.48 mg	0.03 mg
Azuki beans	21.2	4.6	2.41 mg	0.03 mg
Fava/faba beans	19.9	5.0	2.26 mg	0.57 mg
Great northern beans	17.7	7.2	2.01 mg	0.82 mg

Adapted from Kaufman PB, et al. A comparative survey of leguminous plants as sources of the isoflavones genistein and daidzein: implications for human nutrition and health. *J Alt Compl Med* 3(1): 7–12, 1997 is processing.[42] A recent analysis found a reduction in isoflavones in soymilk, which is not a particularly good source of isoflavones anyway.[43] Regular soymilk contains 53.2 mg genistein per liter, while low-fat soymilk contains 24.2 mg, and nonfat contains 6.5 mg. Tofu, a much better source of isoflavones, showed some depletion of daidzein (133.1 mcg/g in regular versus 98.9 mcg/g in low-fat) but only a trivial drop in genistein (169.0 mcg/g in regular versus 153.2 mcg/g in low-fat).

Some people prefer the seeming simplicity of getting their isoflavones from supplements. There are no studies of humans on the long-term effects from large doses of dietary supplements that contain purified isoflavones such as genistein or daidzein, and it is unclear whether heavy intake of phytoestrogens in postmenopausal breast cancer patients is beneficial or harmful. What's more, there is no data available on the interactions that may occur when supplemental phytoestrogens are used concurrently with tamoxifen or raloxifene.

Summary

We believe that phytoestrogens from food sources are safe and beneficial to the health of premenopausal women and that they can alleviate menopausal symptoms in postmenopausal women. The safety of supplemental phytoestrogens in postmenopausal women with breast cancer is not clearly established.

CHAPTER EIGHT

Herbs

A Mixed Bag

Many women use herbs to relieve menopausal symptoms. Although several herbs have a long history of use, their efficacy and safety are not established in clinical studies.

At forty-nine, Sara Altschul, a magazine editor noted for her funny jokes and wild sense of humor, was nonplussed to find that every time she cracked a joke during a meeting, her normally fair skin blushed bright red.

"It was unbelievably embarrassing," says Sara. "It never used to happen. Then it dawned on me that I was having these blushes three or four times a day. And it hit me—*these* must be hot flashes!"

Sara wanted to take herbs during menopause, and she started with black cohosh. "Within two or three weeks my hot flashes disappeared," she says. "I took it regularly for two or three months. Then I went on vacation and stopped taking it."

She shrugs. "The hot flashes never returned."

Power Herbs

When menopausal symptoms start to interfere with life, many women use herbs to relieve them. Black cohosh, chaste-tree berry, dong quai, ginkgo, ginseng, kava, licorice, red clover, and St. John's wort are among the most popular.

Unfortunately, clinical studies on the efficacy and safety of these herbs are lacking, even though some of them have powerful hormone-like effects.

Here are the most commonly used herbs—and what we know about them so far.

Black Cohosh (*Cimicifuga racemosa*)

The roots and rhizomes (underground stems) of black cohosh contain alkaloids, including *N*-methylcytisine, terpenoids, cimicifugin, salicylic acid, and tannins. We're not sure whether they contain phytoestrogens, which are naturally occurring plant estrogens.

> Unfortunately, clinical studies on the efficacy and safety of these herbs are lacking, even though some of them have powerful hormone-like effects.

Three studies showed improvement in menopausal symptoms in women who took black cohosh.[1, 2, 3] The studies made use of the Kupperman Menopausal Symptom Index, a long-used but inadequate scale of menopausal symptoms. Two obvious examples of its inadequacy: It does not include vaginal dryness, but it does include formication, or the sensation of insects crawling on one's body.

The only study to report on hot flashes as a separate symptom was the Stoll trial. It found that hot flashes decreased more in the black cohosh group than in the placebo group.[4] Another recent trial in breast cancer survivors found no relief from hot flashes.

While all trials used the standardized black cohosh product, Remifemin, the formulation has changed over the years from a liquid to tablets, and the dosage of extract in each tablet has also increased from 2 mg to 20 mg. Both factors make it difficult to compare earlier studies with those using the dose and form recommended today.

A recent randomized, double-blind, placebo-controlled trial in eighty-five breast cancer survivors (sixty-nine of whom completed it), found that while black cohosh did not reduce hot flashes more than placebo, it significantly lessened excessive sweating. Women took one tablet twice daily of a placebo or black cohosh (apparently 20 mg of Remifemin) for two months. This study, by Jacobson, measured hot flashes, excessive sweating, palpitations, headaches, poor sleep, depression, and irritability.[5]

Fifty-nine of the women were also taking tamoxifen. The frequency and intensity of hot flashes decreased in both groups, but there was no statistical difference between the black cohosh and the placebo group. Excessive sweating decreased significantly more in the treatment group than in the placebo group. Other symptoms improved equally in both groups. Scores on a health and well-being scale did not change in either group.

An unblinded, controlled, three-month comparative study compared forty drops of Remifemin liquid twice a day with conjugated estrogens at the standard dosage of 0.625 mg per day and diazepam (a tranquilizer) at 2 mg per day.[6] In sixty women ages forty-five to sixty with menopausal complaints, the Kupperman Index, the Hamilton Anxiety Scale, the Self-Assessment Depression Scale, and the Clinical Global Impression Scale improved with all therapies—although it is not clear how much improvement actually occurred. The authors concluded that Remifemin was at least as effective as estrogen and better than diazepam.

Next was a double-blind, placebo-controlled, three-month trial of 4 mg of Remifemin taken twice a day versus conjugated estrogens, again at the standard 0.625 mg per day, and a placebo. The subjects were eighty menopausal women (seventy-five of them completed the study) ages forty-six to fifty-six who had more than three hot flashes a day and mood complaints. The study found that the Kupperman Index, the Hamilton Scale, and vaginal lubrication significantly improved in the Remifemin group (p<0.001). There was no change in the estrogen or placebo groups.[7] Hot flashes decreased from 4.9 to 0.7 in the Remifemin group; from 5.2 to 3.2 in the estrogen group; and from 5.1 to 3.1 in the placebo group.

Last was a randomized, controlled six-month trial of sixty women under age forty who'd had hysterectomies and retained at least one ovary and were having menopausal symptoms. The study tested the effects of 4 mg of Remifemin taken twice a day versus estriol at

1 mg per day versus conjugated estrogens at 1.25 mg per day versus an estrogen/progesterone combination.[8] The Kupperman Index, modified to seventeen symptoms, improved in all groups.

Uterine Effects   It's unclear whether black cohosh is estrogenic. This is important to know, because estrogens can stimulate abnormal endometrial growth and are associated with endometrial cancer.

No human studies have adequately evaluated the effect of black cohosh on uterine endometrium. Two German studies found no effect of black cohosh extract (Remifemin 136 mg per day in one study, an unspecified extract in another) on uterine endometrium after three months.[9] However, three months is too short a time to see estrogenic effects on endometrium. Laboratory tests and animal tests on the estrogenic effect of black cohosh are not consistent.

Black Cohosh in Breast Cancer Survivors   The Jacobson study found that black cohosh had no effect on hot flashes in women who had breast cancer, and it's not known whether this herb is safe for breast cancer survivors. Laboratory tests of black cohosh on breast cancer cells have been mixed.[10] One recent study found that black cohosh significantly increased the growth of breast cancer cells compared with untreated control cells (an effect similar to that of estrogen 17 ß-estradiol).[11] A constituent of black cohosh, fukinolic acid, increased growth of breast cancer cells; again, the effect was similar to estradiol.[12]

How It Works   Actually, we don't know how black cohosh works. We don't know whether it contains phyto-estrogens. Formononetin, an estrogenic isoflavone, was isolated from black cohosh extract in one study,[13] while another study found no formononetin.[14] The recently identified fukinolic acid may be a new phytoestrogen. There are no available data indicating which compounds in black cohosh are responsible for its beneficial effects.

Recommendation   There is no published study in which black cohosh has been taken for longer than six months. This concerns us, because women using this product for hot flashes or as "natural" hormone replacement therapy may take it for years.

There are also no published human studies on long-term safety, particularly regarding endometrial or breast stimulation, and laboratory studies are not consistent or sufficient. While black cohosh seems to be a useful herb for menopausal symptoms, we cannot presume it is safe for long-term use until appropriate studies are conducted. Side effects of black cohosh include frontal headache, stomach discomfort, nausea, vomiting, disturbances in vision, and possibly a slow heartbeat.

Commission E, part of the German agency that is equivalent to the U.S. Food and Drug Administration, does not recommend using black cohosh for longer than six months. We agree with this caution. Although there are no reported cases of endometrial cancer associated with use of black cohosh, we are concerned about the risk of endometrial cancer with long-term use.

Use of estrogens without progestins increases endometrial cancer risk, and if there are estrogens in black cohosh, they may not be entirely safe. Phytoestrogens present in herbs are not the same as those present in food plants such as soybeans and whole grains, and they may not be as benign.

In summary, black cohosh is an herb that helps relieve menopausal symptoms but that should not be used for longer than six months until the safety of longer term use is determined. Although there is some evidence for its effectiveness, there are few studies of acceptable scientific caliber.

> Use of estrogens without progestins increases endometrial cancer risk, and if there are estrogens in black cohosh, they may not be entirely safe.

The usual dose of black cohosh is 0.3 to 2.0 grams in capsules or infusion three times a day; liquid extract (1:1 herb to solvent ratio in 90 percent alcohol) 0.3 to 2.0 ml each day; tincture (1:10 in 60 percent alcohol) 2 to 4 ml each day; or tablets (40 mg standardized extract once a day). Although black cohosh is available in ointments and salves, no one is sure whether our skin actually absorbs it.

Chaste-Tree Berry (*Vitex agnus-castus*)

Chaste-tree berry, also called vitex, contains flavonoids (primarily casticin) and iridoids (aucubin and agnuside). Scientists don't yet know what the most active compounds are. There have been no clinical studies on vitex for menopausal symptoms, although many herbalists believe that it "balances" hormone levels, especially in women with unpredictable or heavy bleeding before menopause.

> There have been no clinical studies on vitex for menopausal symptoms, although many herbalists believe that it "balances" hormone levels, especially in women with unpredictable or heavy bleeding before menopause.

Scientists don't know what effect this herb has on postmenopausal women. The herb is called chaste-tree berry and monk's pepper because it is reputed to lower libido in both women and men.

The usual dose is 0.5 to 1.0 grams of the fruit three times a day or aqueous-alcohol extracts corresponding to 30 to 40 mg of the crushed fruits.

Recommendation   Chaste-tree berry is a relatively benign herb. It may cause an acne-like rash or itching in some people, but really severe adverse effects have not been reported. There are no clinical trials on its use for menopausal symptoms, but it appears to be safe.

Dong Quai (*Angelica sinensis*)

Dong quai is a Chinese herb commonly prescribed for menopausal women. It contains no known phytoestrogens. One double-blind, placebo-controlled study of seventy-one postmenopausal women found that this herb by itself did not affect the number of hot flashes, estrogenization of vaginal cells, or endometrial thickness as measured by sonogram.[15] Keep in mind, however, that Chinese herbs are generally used in mixtures rather than by themselves. The usual dose is 3 to 10 grams of sliced dried root per day or as a liquid extract (1:1, 25 percent ethanol): 0.5 to 2 ml three times daily. Dong quai contains anticoagulant coumarins[16] and can cause bleeding when administered concurrently with warfarin (commonly known by the brand name Coumadin) or, potentially, other anticoagulants.[17] It also contains furocoumarins, which can cause easy sunburning (photosensitization).[18]

Siberian Ginseng or Eleuthero (*Eleutherococcus senticosus*)

Siberian "ginseng" is not ginseng at all, although both it and *Panax ginseng*—the real ginseng—are in the same family. Both are tonic, adaptogenic herbs and are used for some of the same purposes. There are no studies on the use of eleuthero to treat menopausal women.

The usual dose is 0.6 to 3 grams daily of dry root or 0.5 to 6.0 ml of an alcohol extract daily for up to a month. After a month, a two- to three-week break is usually recommended before using the herb again.

Evening Primrose (*Oenethera biennis*)

Evening primrose oil, an expensive but good source of linoleic and gamma linolenic acid, has been evaluated in a double-blind controlled trial of fifty-six women and found to be no more effective than a placebo for hot flashes.[19] The usual dose is 3 to 8 grams daily (six to sixteen 500 mg capsules).

Ginkgo (Ginkgo biloba)

Ginkgo contains a variety of compounds. Reputed to increase blood flow through small vessels, including cerebral arteries, ginkgo acts as an antioxidant and blood thinner.

In humans, side effects are rare. The most serious problem is bleeding. In five reports of bleeding, most of the patients were receiving anticoagulant drugs at the same time they were taking the ginkgo.[20] Based on this, we think ginkgo extracts should probably be avoided by patients with hemophilia or who are taking anticoagulants. Other side effects include nausea, headache, stomach problems, diarrhea, allergy, anxiety, or sleep disturbances.

A recent summary of all published articles in which ginkgo was given for dementia shows it may be helpful in early Alzheimer's disease.[21] The trials included in the analysis were randomized, double-blind, and placebo-controlled. The analysis excluded patients with depression or other neurologic disease, excluded use of other central nervous system–active medications, included use of standardized ginkgo extract at any dose, had at least one outcome measure that was an objective assessment of cognitive function, and contained sufficient statistical information for meta-analysis.

While the researchers looked at more than fifty articles, they eliminated most of them because there was a lack of clear diagnoses of dementia and Alzheimer's. In four studies that met all inclusion criteria, a total of 212 subjects participated in each of the placebo and ginkgo treatment groups. Overall, there was a significant effect ($p<0.0001$) that translated into a 3 percent difference in the Alzheimer's Disease Assessment Scale for cognition. The authors concluded that ginkgo has a small but significant effect at a dosage of 120 to 240 mg when it is taken for three to six months.

> A recent summary of all published articles in which ginkgo was given for dementia shows it may be helpful in early Alzheimer's disease.

A recent twenty-four-week, randomized, double-blind, placebo-controlled trial of older persons with mild to moderate Alzheimer's disease or vascular dementia (sixty-three were demented), or age-associated memory impairment, tested the effects of a standardized ginkgo extract, EGb 761, in two doses (either 240 or 160 mg per day) against placebo for twenty-four weeks.[22] After twelve weeks of treatment, the initial ginkgo users were re-randomized either to continue ginkgo or to switch to the placebo. Those initially assigned to the placebo continued on it for another twelve weeks.

Measures included neuropsychological testing, verbal learning, clinical assessment of geriatric symptoms, depressive mood, self-perceived health and memory status, and behavioral assessment.

The outcome measures showed no effect for the seventy-nine people who took ginkgo compared with the forty-four who took the placebo for the twenty-four-week period. At the time of the twelve-week assessment, the ginkgo groups (166 people) performed slightly better with regard to self-reported activities of daily life, but slightly worse with regard to self-perceived health status compared with the placebo group of forty-eight people.

Ginkgo did not produce any serious adverse events. This new study differs from previous studies, but the older studies were of longer duration (six to twelve months). A simple explanation is that ginkgo may work best as a preventative agent than as treatment.

Ginkgo may help relieve forgetfulness and other less specific symptoms. A double-blind study of thirty-one patients over age fifty with mild to moderate memory impairment found a beneficial effect on some but not all other tests of cognitive function.[23]

A meta-analysis of forty controlled trials for "cerebral insufficiency" (a syndrome not recognized as a disease in the United States that includes memory and concentration problems, confusion, fatigue, depression, ringing in the ears, and headache) found in twenty-six studies that the people who took ginkgo did significantly better than those in the control group.

In another thirteen studies, there were benefits for some but not all measurements. Most of the studies are of poor quality, particularly in their methodology. Of the eight well-performed trials, all showed a significant benefit for the people taking ginkgo.[24]

Ginkgo leaf extracts should not be used by those with bleeding problems or those who are on anticoagulants, as ginkgo inhibits platelet function and bleeding complications can occur.[25]

The usual dose is 40 mg standardized extract three times a day.

Ginseng (*Panax ginseng* or *Panax quinquefolius*)

Ginseng is regarded as a tonic or adaptogenic herb in Chinese medicine, which means that it is believed to have the ability to rebalance body chemistry until it more nearly approaches a normal healthy state. Ginseng contains terpenoids, especially a group called ginsenosides.

A standardized ginseng extract was tested in 384 menopausal women in a four-month, randomized, double-blind, placebo-controlled trial.[26] There were no significant differences between groups in the Psychological General Well-Being Index, Women's Health Questionnaire, hot flashes, endometrial thickness, vaginal maturation index, or levels of estradiol, or FSH, a hormone that is higher in postmenopausal women unless they take supplemental estrogen.

Ginseng can cause estrogenic effects, although the plant does not actually contain phytoestrogens. The estrogenic effects became known through several cases of postmenopausal uterine bleeding reported by patients who took it.[27, 28] At least one other case occurred after use of a face cream that contained ginseng.[29]

There are different types of ginseng, including Chinese ginseng (*Panax ginseng*) and American ginseng (*Panax quinquefolius*). All may cause hypertension in some individuals. Also, mastalgia (swollen breasts) was reported in a seventy-year-old woman who had taken ginseng powder for three weeks.[30] The same effect, with nipple enlargement and "increased sexual responsive-ness" was reported in five other cases.[31]

In Chinese medicine, *Panax ginseng* and *Panax quin-quefolius* are not interchangeable and are prescribed for different conditions. Ginseng should not be combined with other stimulants and can interact with warfarin and the antidepressant phenelzine.[32]

The usual dose for long-term use is 0.4 to 0.8 grams of the root daily.

Kava (*Piper methysticum*)

Kava, a psychoactive member of the pepper family, is taken for anxiety and insomnia in both Europe and the United States. It appears to be a safe herb for short-term relief. There have been several placebo-controlled trials that show it significantly reduces anxiety.[33]

> Kava, a psychoactive member of the pepper family, is taken for anxiety and insomnia in both Europe and the United States. It appears to be a safe herb for short-term relief.

There is only one study of kava for menopausal symptoms. Forty women using doses of 30 to 60 mg per day for a minimum of fifty-six days found significant improvements in the Hamilton Anxiety Scale and the Kupperman Index of menopausal symptoms.[34] In a follow-up study of forty women taking 210 mg per day, similar relief from anxiety was reported.[35]

Using Herbs Wisely

Herbs can be powerful medicine. Some women think they're safer than drugs because they're "natural." However, herbs can have pharmacological effects and side effects, too. That's why a hierarchy of caution is in order.

Plants that are used for food are generally safe to consume (see Phytoestrogens on page 73) in food-sized portions. For example, the amount of sage in turkey stuffing is safe, but daily use of sage tea could have toxic effects.

"Adaptogen" herbs or "tonic" herbs such as ginseng have traditional uses for a variety of conditions. They are meant to help strengthen our adaptive capabilities and help us respond to stress. Herbs with a history of long-term use are probably safe, but consultation with a health care provider knowledgeable about herbs is recommended if you are considering long-term use.

Individual herbs used to treat menopausal symptoms such as hot flashes should not be used longer than six months. There is little information on the long-term effects of many of these herbs, including black cohosh. Traditionally, herbs are used for a limited time, and there is no reason to assume that they are safe for long-term use.

Kava can cause mild gastrointestinal upsets or allergic skin reactions. Large chronic doses can cause a fish scale–like skin rash, often accompanied by eye irritation. Kava can decrease the effect of levodopa in Parkinson's patients. One case report noted disorientation and lethargy when a patient took kava combined with the benzodiazepine alprazolam, but this person was also on other medications that could have caused the interaction.[36]

The usual dose of kava for anxiety is a standardized extract containing the equivalent of 210 mg of kavalactones daily (usually divided into three doses). For the treatment of menopausal symptoms, the usual dose is 30 to 60 mg kavalactones daily. Kava has recently been linked to liver problems.

Licorice (*Glycyrrhiza glabra*)

The best-known ingredients in licorice are glycyrrhizinic acid and its derivatives.

The herb is reputed to have estrogenic effects; it also has anti-inflammatory properties and increases available levels of cortisol (a steroid hormone made by the adrenal glands that increases when we're stressed). Large or chronic doses may result in swelling, high blood pressure, and low potassium levels that can cause heart arrhythmias. There is one reported case of nonfatal cardiac arrest.[37]

In Chinese medicine, licorice is always used with other ingredients, and the synergistic effects of mixtures as well as dose limitations may prevent problems. All reported cases of licorice-induced problems have been linked to candies, gum, laxatives, or chewing tobacco, not from the use of licorice as herbal medicine. (Most "licorice" candies manufactured in the United States are actually flavored with anise; imported candies usually contain real licorice.)[38]

Because licorice can lower potassium levels, it should not be combined with diuretics. Also, the side effects of licorice can mimic the effects—and side effects—of systemic steroids.

Deglycyrrhizinated forms of licorice are available and recommended for conditions such as ulcers. Glycyrrhizin appears to be the culprit when patients experience serious side effects. However, glycyrrhizin also is the most active compound in licorice, so deglycyrrhizinated licorice may not work as well for some conditions.

There are no clinical trials of licorice for menopausal symptoms. Licorice is not a benign herb, and we do *not* recommend its use to treat menopausal symptoms unless it is part of a mixture prescribed by a traditional practitioner of Chinese medicine.

> Licorice is not a benign herb, and we do *not* recommend its use to treat menopausal symptoms unless it is part of a mixture prescribed by a traditional practitioner of Chinese medicine.

The usual dose is 1 to 4 grams of the root in an infusion (made like tea but steeped for twenty to thirty minutes) or 0.6 to 2.0 grams of licorice extract daily.

Red Clover (*Trifolium pratense*)

Red clover contains the phytoestrogens formononetin, biochanin A, daidzein, and genistein.[39]

Two double-blind, placebo-controlled trials (both funded by Novogen, a manufacturer of red clover extract) have found no benefit for red clover extract. A crossover trial of a standardized product called Promensil (containing 40 mg total isoflavones, including 4 mg of genistein, 3.5 mg of daidzein, 24.5 mg of biochanin, and 8.0 mg of formononetin)[40] enrolled fifty-one women whose last menses was at least six months past and who were having at least three hot flashes a day. They were randomized to one daily tablet of placebo or Promensil.

The first phase of the trial lasted for three months, followed by a one-month washout period, after which the women crossed over to the other treatment for fourteen weeks. (There was an extra two weeks to accommodate for the possibility of a change in reporting habits that might occur at the end of a trial.) Symptom diaries utilizing the Greene Menopause Score (a validated symptom self-assessment scale) were kept by the subjects.

At the beginning of the trial and at the conclusion of each treatment arm, participants underwent a medical examination and blood tests. A vaginal smear was collected for the vaginal maturation index, and transvaginal ultrasound was performed to assess endometrial thickness.

Forty-three women completed the study. Hot flash frequency decreased in both placebo and active groups at twelve weeks (about 18 percent and 20 percent, respectively), but there were no statistically significant differences in Greene Scores between groups at any point. No significant differences were seen between groups in blood tests. Weight did not change in either group. There were no differences between groups in endometrial thickness or vaginal maturation index at the beginning and end of the trial. Urinary isoflavones increased significantly in the Promensil group but not in the placebo group (p<0.001). There appeared to be a correlation between the level of total urinary isoflavones excretion (particularly daidzein) and reduction of hot flashes (regardless of treatment group). Information on adverse events was not reported.

The number of subjects was small, and the efficacy data are not compelling, as no significant effect on hot flashes or Greene Scores were noted. The treatment period was too short to determine conclusively the safety of the product in terms of endometrial stimulation.

Another trial randomized thirty-seven postmenopausal women having at least three hot flashes per day to placebo or one of two doses of Promensil (40 mg or 160 mg) for twelve weeks.[41]

Endpoints were similar to the first trial. Hot flash frequency decreased in all groups over the twelve-week period by 35 percent, 29 percent, and 34 percent. There was no significant difference among the three groups.

> We do not recommend the use of red clover extracts for the treatment of menopausal symptoms. It doesn't seem to work, and it may be unsafe.

There were no significant differences from baseline in any group in follicle-stimulating hormone, sex-hormone-binding globulin, vaginal maturation scores, or vaginal pH (the latter two are biological indicators of estrogenic activity). No "gross abnormalities" in blood counts or liver function tests were reported.

Nowhere in the paper is there a report of adverse events. The paper states, "Two patients were subsequently withdrawn from the 160 mg group because of intervention by their general practitioners," but there is no indication if the intervention was necessary because of adverse effects associated with the treatment.

Traditionally, red clover has not been used long-term or for hot flashes, and it is unknown whether long-term use has an estrogenic effect on the breast or endometrium. Also, the presence of coumarins in some clover species theoretically increases the risk of bleeding, although cases have not been reported.[42, 43]

We do not recommend the use of red clover extracts for the treatment of menopausal symptoms. It doesn't seem to work, and it may be unsafe.

Sage (Salvia officinalis)

Sage is reputed to help hot flashes and night sweats. It contains a volatile oil called thujone, other monoterpenes, and tannins. Thujone is toxic, and long-term use can cause seizures or other neurological symptoms.[44] We do not recommend the use of sage because of its toxicity.

St. John's Wort (Hypericum perforatum)

St. John's wort (SJW) is very popular in the United States as an antidepressant. The studies performed on this herb come from Europe, primarily Germany.

A recent meta-analysis evaluated twenty-three randomized trials (twenty were double-blind) of St. John's wort in a total of 1,757 outpatients with mild to moderate depression.[45] Improvement in depressive symptoms occurred in all groups.

In fifteen placebo-controlled trials, SJW was found to be almost three times better than placebo. In eight treatment-controlled trials, clinical improvement in those receiving SJW did not differ significantly from those receiving tricyclic antidepressants. (It should be noted that the doses of antidepressants in these trials were lower than those normally prescribed in the United States, and there are no trials comparing St. John's wort with the popular selective serotonin reuptake inhibitors Prozac, Zoloft, etc.)

Side effects in these trials were reported less often with SJW than with antidepressants: 19.8 percent of those on SJW reported symptoms, compared with 52.8 percent of those on tricyclic antidepressants.

Other studies indicate that gastrointestinal effects and fatigue may occur with SJW, although easy sunburning may be the most common effect.

Fair-skinned people using SJW should wear sunblock for normal daily sun exposure and should avoid sunbathing. St. John's wort can decrease the effects of tricyclic antidepressants, warfarin, digoxin, theophylline, cyclosporine, indinavir, and other drugs. It may increase the risk of breakthrough bleeding in women on oral contraceptive pills. It increases side effects in those taking selective serotonin reuptake inhibitors.

St. John's wort is a reasonable antidepressant but should not be combined with other antidepressants. In addition, it should not be used by anyone taking daily medication unless the person is under close medical supervision. The usual dose is 300 mg of a preparation standardized to 0.3 percent hypericin or 3 percent hyperforin three times a day.

CHAPTER NINE

"Natural" Hormones

Powerful Friends, Formidable Foes

Hormones, whether synthesized in a lab or manu-factured from natural plant substances, are power-ful, interactive chemicals that affect many parts of the body.

Although hormones can relieve the symptoms of menopause, a risk-free hormone has yet to be invented. We should be very skeptical of any claims that a particular hormone will extend life, reverse aging, restore youth, or prevent dis-ease without causing any adverse effects. If there's one thing we should have learned from the estrogen craze of the 1960s, it's that hormones—whether recommended by a doctor or the cashier at the

> If there's one thing we should have learned from the estrogen craze of the 1960s, it's that hormones are not panaceas. They are powerful drugs that should be treated with respect.

health food store—are not panaceas. They are powerful drugs that should be treated with respect.

Hormonally speaking, there is no free pass.

Here's what we know so far about the "natural" hormones you're most likely to see on the market.

Dehydroepiandrosterone (DHEA)

DHEA is produced by the adrenal glands and is a precursor of both testosterone and estrogen. Marketers tout it as an anti-aging, anticancer miracle supplement, and some natural hormone proponents think it should be added to HRT regimens.

> In the 1950s, estrogen was touted to women as an anti-aging miracle. A decade later we learned that it caused endometrial cancer.

Levels of DHEA-S (a sulfated form of DHEA) in the blood peak at twenty to twenty-four years of age. Each decade thereafter, they fall to 80 percent of the previous decade's level. Between ages eighty-five and ninety, the DHEA-S level averages about 10 percent of what it was at age twenty.[1]

Proponents use this fact as "evidence" that DHEA is the "fountain of youth." Their theory is that replacing DHEA will reverse aging.

Sound familiar? Risk-free youth serums remain a dream. In the 1950s, estrogen was touted to women as an anti-aging miracle. A decade later we learned that it caused endometrial cancer.

Now, forty years later, in what a cynic might say is a mark of progress for equality of the sexes, DHEA is being touted as a panacea for both men and women. Its effects in men and women are very different, however, and women should view this drug with caution. Although it is available over the counter, it is a powerful steroid hormone and should be treated as such.

Proponents of DHEA point to its anticancer and anticardiovascular disease effects in animals as evidence of its great potential. However, DHEA acts differently in humans. Most animals have low to no circulating DHEA to start with and experience dramatic effects with supplementation. Rodents, for example, have almost undetectable DHEA, and even monkeys have much lower levels than do humans.[2] A spectacular effect in a rat that has never encountered DHEA has limited implications for humans who have plenty of DHEA to begin with.

The Gender Gap

The differing effects DHEA has on men and women have serious implications—especially for women.

For one thing, DHEA increases testosterone levels in women but not men.[3] It also has more androgenic than estrogenic effects in women and can cause acne and increase facial and body hair.

One study found not only that androgen levels (including testosterone and androstenedione) *doubled* in women, but also that HDL (the good cholesterol) decreased significantly.[4] Another study found that DHEA supplementation in women decreases sex-hormone-binding-globulin (SHBG) levels. Since high levels of SHBG are associated with lower risks of breast cancer, this effect is just the opposite of what women need.[5] In men, high levels of DHEA-S seem to correlate with less cardiovascular disease,[6, 7] but in women, high levels seem to correlate with increased risk.[8]

Breast and Ovarian Cancer

Different levels of DHEA may have different implications for women of different ages. Premenopausal breast cancer patients seem to have lower levels of DHEA-S than do their peers without breast cancer,[9, 10] but postmenopausal breast cancer patients have higher levels.[11, 12]

A study comparing serum levels of hormones in stored blood from thirty-one women later diagnosed with ovarian cancer and sixty-two other women in a control group found that those who developed ovarian cancer had higher levels of DHEA plus another androgen called androstenedione. In this study, the higher the levels of DHEA and androstenedione, the higher the risk of ovarian cancer.[13]

All of these studies merely found associations and do not prove cause and effect. It's a big jump from noting that men with naturally occurring low DHEA levels have higher rates of cardiovascular disease to concluding that taking DHEA supplements can reduce the risk. It could be, for example, that cardiovascular disease lowers DHEA levels in men rather than that low DHEA levels cause cardiovascular disease.

Nevertheless, these associations raise questions about DHEA supplementation in women. Could taking DHEA as a supplement increase risk for cardiovascular disease and cancer? We urge caution until more research has been done.

Vaginal Thinning

DHEA may help reduce the vaginal thinning that occurs after menopause. In one study, fourteen postmenopausal women tested DHEA in a 10 percent cream for twelve months. The hormone appeared to have marked estrogenic effects on the vaginal cells of almost all the women in the study and did not cause increased growth of the endometrium.[14] Serum lipids were not significantly affected by the DHEA cream.

Effects on Bone

A double-blind, placebo-controlled, randomized trial of twenty-one women (nineteen of them completed the study) with lupus tested the effect of 200 mg a day of DHEA for six months as an adjunct to conventional lupus medications. Women in the DHEA group maintained their bone density levels, while the placebo group experienced significant reduction.[15]

In the trial of DHEA cream mentioned earlier, the application of DHEA in a 10 percent cream to fourteen postmenopausal women for twelve months resulted in significantly increased bone mineral density at the hip.[16]

Mood/Depression

In a placebo-controlled crossover trial of 50 mg of DHEA taken nightly for six months by thirteen men and seventeen women (eight of the women were also using HRT) between the ages of forty and seventy, men and women reported an increased feeling of well being.[17]

Another study that looked at mood and well being found no effect. This was a double-blind, placebo-controlled, randomized trial that tested 50 mg per day of DHEA for three months in sixty perimenopausal women with altered mood and sense of well being.[18] At the end of the trial, the groups did not differ in severity of perimenopausal symptoms, mood, dysphoria, libido, cognition, memory, or well being. Compared to the placebo group, the DHEA group experienced an increase in DHEA and testosterone and a decrease in cortisol levels.

Yet another study was a double-blind, placebo-controlled six-week trial of DHEA (up to 90 mg per day) in twenty-two patients with major depression. The patients were either medication free or on stabilized antidepressant regimens. The study found that those who took DHEA had a significantly greater decrease in the Hamilton Depression Rating Scale than those in the placebo group. Five of eleven DHEA-treated patients (compared with one out of eleven in the placebo group) experienced a 50 percent decrease in depressive symptoms.[19]

A double-blind, randomized crossover trial in seventeen men and women with midlife-onset dysthymia (a type of depression) compared two doses of DHEA (90 mg and 450 mg, each for three weeks) with placebo for six weeks.[20] Sixty percent of the DHEA-treated group, compared with 20 percent of the placebo-treated group, cut their depression symptoms in half, as measured on either the Hamilton Scale or the Beck Depression Inventory. There was no difference between groups in terms of cognitive tests or sleep disturbances.

Cognition

In a double-blind crossover study of forty healthy elderly men and women given 50 mg of DHEA for two weeks, there was no effect on psychological or cognitive parameters.[21] DHEA, androstenedione, and testosterone increased in both men and women in this study. Another placebo-controlled trial by the same investigator in thirty-six younger men tested a single dose of DHEA at 300 mg and found no significant difference in memory performance.[22]

Body Composition

While some smaller studies show mixed results on the effect of DHEA on body composition, larger, blinded studies show no benefit.

In a double-blind crossover trial, the thirty subjects (ages forty to seventy) included seventeen women. They took 50 mg a day of DHEA for three months and neither men nor women had any change in percentage of body fat or body mass index.[23]

In a randomized, double-blind, placebo-controlled trial, morbidly obese adolescents took 40 mg of DHEA twice a day for eight weeks.[24] There was no effect on body weight, body composition, serum lipids, or insulin sensitivity, but the females' testosterone levels increased significantly.

An uncontrolled study of fifteen healthy post-menopausal women showed decreases in skin fold measurements of 9.8 percent, an increase in the midthigh muscular area of 3.5 percent, and decreased femoral fat of 3.8 percent after twelve months when the subjects rubbed a 10 percent DHEA cream into their skin.[25] Plasma sex-hormone-binding-globulin, the "good" HDL cholesterol, and total cholesterol decreased, as did fasting glucose and fasting insulin levels. Skin also got oilier. Measurements returned to baseline within three months of discontinuing DHEA.

> DHEA is a potent hormonal drug. As an anti-aging supplement or a new version of HRT, however, we have not seen sufficient evidence to recommend it.

Summary

DHEA is a potent hormonal drug. In high doses it may increase bone density, lift depression, and treat other conditions. As an anti-aging supplement or a new version of HRT, however, we have not seen sufficient evidence to recommend it.

Although there is preliminary evidence that DHEA may decrease vaginal dryness and increase bone density, using DHEA supplements may also cause increased body hair and acne in women, and there are unanswered safety concerns about a possible increased risk of cardiovascular disease or cancer.

DHEA should be regarded as a powerful drug, not a dietary supplement. It may be useful as treatment for lupus and other medical conditions when used under a doctor's supervision.

Estriol

Some are pushing estriol by itself or in tri-estrogen mixtures as a safer form of HRT. It is touted as a "good" estrogen that does not cause endometrial or breast cancer. Some even claim that it prevents breast cancer, although there is no scientific evidence to back this up.

Estriol is a weak estrogen that can be used to treat menopausal symptoms, including hot flashes, if menopausal women take it in high doses.[26, 27] It also seems to be beneficial in maintaining bone mineral density.[28, 29]

Some practitioners of alternative medicine promote the mixture tri-estrogen, or tri-est, which contains estrone, estradiol, and estriol. Typically, the proportions are 80 percent estriol, 10 percent estrone, and 10 percent estradiol, and the practitioners usually recommend doses of 2.5 to 5 mg a day either continuously or for twenty-five days a month. Natural progesterone cream is often prescribed with this regimen, although progesterone creams are not absorbed well enough to protect the uterus from estrogen's effects.

Estriol or estriol mixtures are not commonly used by conventional medical practitioners in the United States. Proponents claim that estriol has anticancer effects in animals, that low estriol levels are associated with breast cancer, and that estriol does not cause endometrial stimulation. All of these claims arise from a handful of poor studies done in the 1970s, almost all of them by one person, Henry Lemon. Let's take a look at them.

Breast Cancer

The first study we'll examine was published in 1966 and included fifty-seven premenopausal and postmenopausal subjects with breast cancer and forty-one without breast cancer. The study reports that the women with breast cancer excreted 30 to 60 percent less estriol per twenty-four hours than did the women used as controls.[30] However, these results were not statistically significant. The study states, "The differences between the group means for estriol excretion alone, or for the mean or median Eq values between the two groups, did not attain the 5 percent confidence level by various parametrical and non-parametrical tests."

"Eq" stands for "estriol excretion quotient," a ratio of estriol to estrone and estradiol. This is an unconventional test, apparently invented by the authors. The authors' conclusion is based entirely on this higher number of "subnormal" Eq among breast cancer patients compared with controls in a subanalysis. The authors don't define "subnormal." Results on an unvalidated test count for nothing.

In addition, there is reason to suspect that a number of women in the control group may have had abnormal ovarian function that could have affected results: Nine of twenty-four premenopausal women in the control group were infertile, two of ten postmenopausal controls had "other cancers," and three had "polycystic ovaries or cortical fibrosis."

In a later article, the same author cites three studies (including the one just mentioned) as evidence for reduced estriol excretion in breast cancer and cites seven studies that found no difference.[31] Although he notes that "initial reports of reduced estriol excretion in breast carcinoma have not been substantiated by others,"[32] he continues to argue that estriol may be useful in breast cancer prevention.[33, 34] This is particularly notable, since by his own report six of twenty-four breast cancer patients treated with 5 to 15 mg of estriol daily experienced "increased growth of metastases," and two developed endometrial hyperplasia. Five others also experienced vaginal bleeding.[35]

We often hear estriol proponents say a study has shown that estriol arrested metastasis or caused remission of breast cancer in 37 percent of patients. They are referring to a commentary by Follingstad that contains a quote from an unpublished study by Lemon, in which an unspecified number of postmenopausal breast cancer patients received between 2.5 and 15 mg of estriol for an unspecified amount of time.[36] The study itself explicitly states that its purpose was to test safety, not efficacy.

> Different doses of estrogens have different effects on breast cancer growth: Low doses can stimulate growth, while high doses can inhibit it.

We do know that different doses of estrogens have different effects on breast cancer growth: Low doses can stimulate growth, while high doses can inhibit it. An animal study often quoted by estriol proponents claims that estriol reduces the incidence of breast cancer in rats treated with carcinogens. However, the study actually shows that *all* of the four estrogens tested reduced the incidence of carcinogen-induced breast cancer.[37]

Endometrial Hyperplasia and Cancer

Claims that estriol does not cause endometrial hyperplasia (abnormal growth of cells in the uterine lining that can lead to endometrial cancer) come from a 1978 study that found estriol in a dose of 2 to 8 mg per day improved hot flashes in fifty-two symptomatic menopausal women.[38] Endometrial biopsy showed no evidence of endometrial hyperplasia after six months. Six months, however, is not really long enough to demonstrate endometrial hyperplasia.

In any case, two recent studies show that estriol does cause endometrial stimulation. In one, twenty-nine postmenopausal women scheduled for hysterectomies were treated with 0.5 mg of vaginal estriol daily or 0.05 mg of 17 ß-estradiol daily.[39] Signs of estrogenic stimulation were found in the endometrium (uterine lining), myometrium (uterine muscle), and vagina. Estriol and estradiol had a similar effect. A very large Swedish study of 1,110 women with postmenopausal bleeding found that endometrial hyperplasia was significantly more common in women taking estriol than in women taking sequential estrogen and progestin therapy or in women not receiving HRT.[40]

Summary

Estriol is one of several hormones that some women use to treat hot flashes and other menopausal symptoms. However, there is no reasonable scientific evidence that estriol has anticancer effects or that it is safer than estradiol or conjugated estrogens. If the woman using it has a uterus, she should also take an oral form of progestin to protect the uterus from estrogen-induced endometrial cancer.

Melatonin

Melatonin is a hormone that regulates our daily wake-sleep cycles. It's produced mostly by the pineal gland at the base of the brain and in the intestines, where its production appears to be controlled by nutritional factors—especially the availability of the amino acid tryptophan, a precursor.[41]

Melatonin levels increase when we sleep. The increase is lessened by the presence of even small amounts of light, such as a streetlight shining through a window. Alcohol consumption also blunts melatonin surges, which may be one reason why alcohol causes sleep disturbances.[42] Some scientists think that nightly surges of melatonin may have a beneficial effect in reducing the risk of certain cancers, but this theory has not yet been proven.

There is some evidence that melatonin helps jet lag, sleep quality, and workers' tolerance for working night shifts or varying shifts. There's no evidence that it retards aging. This concept is based on the same fallacy as hormone replacement therapy: You're as young as your hormones, and boosting hormones to youthful levels will provide the health or vigor of youth. Although currently available over the counter, melatonin is a powerful hormone that has a pronounced effect on reproductive hormones. Melatonin receptors are in many parts of the body. Science does not yet know its long-term effects.

A dose range from 0.1 to 3.0 mg best mimics natural body levels. Melatonin can cause sleepiness, headache, lightheadedness or fuzziness, and can worsen depression in some people.

Summary

No information is available about the long-term effects of taking melatonin every night, but occasional use for jet lag or insomnia is probably harmless.

We do not support the daily use of supplemental melatonin as an anti-aging supplement or cancer prophylactic. Although there is intriguing preliminary evidence for the benefits of a nightly melatonin surge, it is not clear that taking pills replicates naturally occurring conditions, and in any case the appropriate dose is unknown.

> There is some evidence that melatonin helps jet lag, sleep quality, and workers' tolerance for working night shifts or varying shifts. There's no evidence that it retards aging.

For those who want to stimulate their natural melatonin, there's certainly no harm in attempting to increase melatonin levels by sleeping in a completely dark room or using a sleep mask.

Natural Progesterone

"Natural progesterone," or micronized progesterone is derived from precursors in soybeans (*Glycine max*) or an inedible Mexican wild yam (*Diascorea villosa*).

The oral form is used in conventional medicine. The sublingual and cream forms are touted by marketers as a prophylactic against hot flashes, osteoporosis, PMS, fibrocystic breasts, and even breast cancer. Almost all these claims started in a popular booklet written by John M. Lee, M.D. Lee claims that the unifying factor linking all of these different conditions is "estrogen dominance secondary to a relative insufficiency of progesterone."[43] Lee also claims that natural progesterone has none of the side effects of the synthetics.

Only the claim that progesterone can help hot flashes has some evidence behind it. In fact, in conventional medicine, oral progestins are sometimes used to treat hot flashes, and one trial supports the use of topical progesterone cream for this purpose. That's it. There is no credible evidence that the treatment benefits bone. Also, we don't absorb enough progesterone from skin creams to prevent estrogen-induced endometrial hyperplasia.

The evidence for a beneficial effect of natural progesterone cream on bone appears in an uncontrolled, unselected, and poorly documented case series.[44] By contrast, a randomized, double-blind, placebo-controlled trial found no effect of progesterone cream on bone. Hot flashes, however, did improve.[45]

In that study, 102 healthy postmenopausal women who were within five years of menopause and not taking hormones applied one-quarter teaspoon of progesterone cream (20 mg of progesterone) or placebo daily. All women also took daily multivitamins and calcium (1200 mg daily). At the end of one year, there were no significant differences between the treatment and control groups in bone mineral density (lumbar spine, femoral neck, or total hip) nor in the number of subjects in each group who showed an increase of bone mineral density of more than 1.2 percent.

Of those who reported hot flashes at the beginning, five of twenty-six women in the control group reported "improvement," in comparison with twenty-five out of thirty women in the treatment group, a significant difference (p<0.001). No significant changes occurred in cholesterol levels or mood ratings in either group, but eight women in the progesterone group experienced vaginal spotting. Postmenopausal bleeding is worrisome because it can indicate endometrial hyperplasia; biopsies should have been done to evaluate this.

Breast Cancer

While oral progestins clearly protect the endometrium from estrogen-induced endometrial cancer, they do not protect the breast.[46]

Epidemiological studies have not shown an increased risk of breast cancer among women using contraceptives that contain only progestin.[47] On the other hand, observational studies indicate that HRT may increase breast cancer risk, and progestins do not appear to decrease this risk.[48] All of this is controversial: The progestin component of HRT has variously been reported to increase, decrease, or not affect breast cancer risk.[49]

Wild Yams and Diosgenin

Soybeans, Mexican wild yams, and other plants (not including the sweet potatoes and yams that we eat) contain diosgenin, the chemical compound from which progesterone is derived.

Bear in mind, there's a lengthy process in a chemistry lab involved in this conversion that our bodies cannot mimic. Despite this, there are now dozens of topical and vaginal preparations sold as "wild yam" creams.

Oral wild yam preparations are used medicinally, primarily to treat gastrointestinal cramping. It is unclear if any active components of wild yam can be absorbed through the skin, but whether or not they are, eating or applying wild yam extract or diosgenin will not result in increased progesterone levels in humans because we cannot convert diosgenin into progesterone. Products that say they contain natural progesterone or progesterone derived from wild yams may actually contain the drug progesterone.

Although derived from a plant, it's as much of a stretch to consider natural progesterone an herbal product as it would be to consider the birth control pill (whose genesis is the same plant) an herbal product. If a product claims to contain only wild yam extract or diosgenin but causes progestin-like effects, then it is mislabeled and actually contains progesterone. If it does contain progesterone, we still don't know how much of it is in the product or how much we will absorb.

Two studies indicate that serum levels of progesterone do not rise high enough after application of skin creams to prevent estrogenic stimulation of the endometrium.

The *Lancet* published a crossover study that compared plasma progesterone and metabolites (breakdown products) after topical application of Pro-Gest cream (one brand of topical progesterone), topical application of placebo, and oral progesterone.[50] Twenty surgically menopausal women who were not taking hormone replacement therapy were randomly assigned to apply one teaspoon of Pro-Gest cream (this is two to four times the recommended daily dose) or a placebo cream twice daily for ten days. There was a four-day washout period, and then the women switched creams. Each subject then took oral progesterone (100 mg in the morning and 200 mg in the evening) for five days.

Compared with the placebo, Pro-Gest significantly increased plasma progesterone levels. However, after ten days of treatment, median plasma levels were only 2.9 nmol/L, compared with 9.5 nmol/L with oral progesterone—not enough to protect the endometrium from estrogen stimulation. This study also found that although each 2-ounce jar said it contained 930 mg of progesterone, it actually contained 200 mg, one-fifth of the amount claimed.

Both Dr. John Lee and Transitions for Health, the manufacturers of Pro-Gest, wrote letters to the *Lancet* after the study was published. Transitions for Health stated that the product contained the proper amount of progesterone and called the study results into question.[51] John Lee's letter states that plasma progesterone does not accurately affect bioavailable levels, because it preferentially enters red blood cell membranes. Lee also suggests that saliva levels are more predictive of bioavailable progesterone.[52]

Cooper and Whitehead, authors of the *Lancet* article, responded, "We find it difficult to envisage how progesterone could bind to red blood cells, but not to serum albumin, corticosteroid-binding globulin, and α-1 glycoprotein, and yet be readily released into saliva . . . we remain very concerned about the clinical use of Pro-Gest because of the absence of scientifically valid studies on endometrial protection and bone conservation. Prescription should follow scientific evaluation— not the reverse."

As if that weren't enough to demonstrate how useless these creams are for protecting the uterus, a twelve-week randomized clinical trial of twenty-seven postmenopausal women aged fifty to sixty-five compared the effects of three different doses of micronized progesterone (16 mg, 32 mg, and 64 mg) topical cream used with a transdermal estrogen patch containing 17 ß-estradiol. The estrogen patch was applied once weekly, and each progesterone cream was applied for the latter two weeks of each four-week treatment cycle. Progesterone levels in the blood rose only to 0.6–3.2 nmol/L—not enough to protect the endometrium—and none of the endometrial biopsies showed evidence of a progesterone response.

Summary

Natural progesterone cream may decrease hot flashes, but it does not help osteoporosis and cannot protect the uterus from cancer when a woman is taking estrogen.

Natural progesterone may be better for cholesterol levels than synthetic progesterone in HRT regimens. However, all progestins can cause depression, bloating, and other symptoms. Although proponents of natural progesterone claim that only synthetic progestins cause these symptoms while the natural form alleviates them—there is no evidence that supports this contention.

> More research needs to be done to determine whether natural progesterone has markedly different beneficial or deleterious effects compared with synthetic progestins.

Clearly, more research needs to be done to determine whether natural progesterone has markedly different beneficial or deleterious effects compared with synthetic progestins. Neither wild yam nor diosgenin is converted to progesterone in the body, although scientists can do it in a lab.

Ipriflavone

Ipriflavone (IP), a relatively benign synthetic drug marketed as a dietary supplement, is heavily promoted for preventing and treating osteoporosis. Although several trials indicate that ipriflavone increases spinal and wrist bone density, no trials have examined bone density at the hip, where the most serious fractures occur. Also, no trials of adequate size have examined nonvertebral fractures. This section will review controlled trials of ipriflavone in naturally or surgically menopausal women.

Effect on Fractures

The most recent, largest, and best randomized, placebo-controlled trial enrolled 474 postmenopausal women who took 200 mg of ipriflavone three times daily for three years. All subjects also received 500 mg of calcium per day. The bone density of the spine, hip, and forearm was assessed by DEXA scan every three months. Markers of bone metabolism in the urine were also assessed. There was no difference between the groups in vertebral fracture rates or bone mineral density at any of the sites. However, lymphocyte concentrations—lymphocytes are a type of white cell—decreased significantly in ipriflavone-treated women, and twenty-nine women developed lymphopenia (low lymphocyte counts). After the ipriflavone was stopped, 48 percent of the women had normal lymphocyte counts after one year and 71 percent returned to normal after two years.

Two small, problematic studies have looked at vertebral fracture rates. Both studies were double-blind, placebo-controlled studies of women over age sixty-five with vertebral fractures. Treated groups received 200 mg of ipriflavone three times a day; all women also received 1 gram of calcium per day.

The first study appeared in the Italian *Journal of Mineral Electrolyte Research*.[53] Only twenty-seven of forty-nine women completed the trial, a very high dropout rate. The treated group experienced an increase in wrist bone mineral density, while the placebo group was unchanged; the difference between the groups was significant at years one and two.

A secondary source on this study states that four out of twenty people in the treatment group had new vertebral fractures, compared with eight out of twenty in the placebo group.[54] This secondary source doesn't state whether this is significant, nor does it state when this occurred.

In the second two-year, randomized, double-blind study of one hundred women (eighty-four women completed it) over age sixty-five with osteoporosis and at least one previous vertebral fracture, researchers compared ipriflavone at 200 mg three times daily with a placebo. All received 1 gram of calcium daily.[55] A significant increase in wrist bone mineral density occurred in the treated group while a significant decrease occurred in the placebo group. Differences between groups were significant at six, twelve, and twenty-four months. Two new vertebral fractures occurred in the treated group, and eleven new vertebral fractures occurred in the placebo group (it is not stated how many patients this represents nor whether this was statistically significant). Analgesic use decreased significantly in the IP group while it increased in the placebo group.

Bone Density in Menopausal Women

In a two-year, double-blind, randomized, controlled trial in multiple locations in Italy, researchers enrolled 255 postmenopausal women aged fifty to sixty-five. IP 200 mg three times daily with meals was compared with a placebo.[56] Both groups also received 1 gram of elemental calcium daily. Bone mineral density at the wrist was measured at baseline and every six months.

Nearly two hundred women completed the trial. According to an intention-to-treat analysis (an analysis including all subjects, based on assigned treatment, even if they did not complete the full course) after two years, the treated group maintained wrist bone density, while the control group's bone density declined; the difference between the two groups was significant at both one and two years.

A paper by Gennari and Adami, also published in 1997, reported the results of two multicenter studies; however, one of these is clearly a republication of the study cited previously.[57] The other study enrolled 198 women, and entry criteria, treatment, duration, and analysis appeared identical to the study just described. However, BMD measurements were taken at the spine and dual energy X-ray absorptiometry (DXA) was used. These factors make this a better study. DXA is a better modality for measuring bone mineral density, which is site-specific—wrist-bone mineral density is not useful for predicting fracture risk at other sites.

The placebo group lost 1.1 percent vertebral bone mineral density at year two, while there were no changes from baseline in the ipriflavone-treated group. It is not stated whether the between-group difference was significant.

Another two-year study enrolled fifty-six post-menopausal Caucasian women with vertebral bone density (measured by DXA) one notch below the

age-matched mean and at least two other risk factors—
low calcium intake, smoking, alcohol or caffeine "abuse,"
sedentary life style, or "familiarity with osteoporosis,"
which presumably means family history. Subjects were
randomized to ipriflavone (200 mg three times daily) or
placebo; both groups also received 1,000 mg of calcium.[58]

Forty out of fifty-six women completed the trial. In
the intention-to-treat analysis, the placebo group lost
bone (–3.8 percent), and the ipriflavone group had no
change (–1.2 percent); the between-group differences
were significant only at year two.

In another study, fifty-seven postmenopausal
women with osteopenia or osteoporosis were randomized to either 600 mg ipriflavone or 0.8 grams per day of
calcium lactate for one year.[59] In the IP group, lumbar
bone mineral density measured by DXA decreased from
0.78 g/cm^2 before treatment to 0.77 g/cm^2 after treatment; in the calcium group, bone mineral density
decreased from 0.81 to 0.79. The authors state that the
rate of reduction of bone mineral density and the
decrease in bone mineral density in comparison to baseline were both significantly greater in the calcium group.
They did not state whether the difference between
groups was significant, but it probably was not.

A double-blind study of forty postmenopausal
women treated with 600 mg of ipriflavone per day or a
placebo (all received 1000 mg of calcium each day) found
that after a year, bone mineral density measured by DXA
in the spine and forearm, compared with baseline, was
significantly reduced in the placebo group, while BMD
was stable in the ipriflavone-treated group.[60]

Ipriflavone and Vitamin D

A study of ipriflavone and vitamin D included ninety-eight postmenopausal, oophorectomized women ages forty-five to sixty-five. Twenty-eight women took 600 mg of ipriflavone daily, fifteen took vitamin D, twenty took both, and thirty-five took neither. No explanation is given for the lopsided allotment. Women were assessed at baseline and every six months for eighteen months. Seventy-nine women completed the study. Vertebral BMD was measured by DXA. All groups lost bone, but the combination of ipriflavone and vitamin D significantly reduced bone loss at all time points compared with all other groups. At eighteen months, the combination group had lost 0.33 percent, the ipriflavone group –2.37 percent, the vitamin D group –1.15 percent, and the control group –3.70 percent.

Ipriflavone and Estrogen

There is some evidence that ipriflavone may be helpful as an adjunct to estrogen in maintaining bone density, but studies are inconsistent. A recent study of 116 Japanese women who'd had their ovaries removed found that ipriflavone alone is inadequate to maintain bone density, although it may be helpful when taken with estrogen. The women were randomized to placebo, 0.625 mg per day of conjugated estrogens, 600 mg per day of ipriflavone, or conjugated estrogens and ipriflavone.[61] At the end of forty-eight weeks, spinal bone mineral density measured by DXA was reduced significantly by 6.1 percent in the placebo group, 3.9 percent in the conjugated estrogen group, and 5.1 percent in the ipriflavone group. There was no significant change in the combined-therapy group where spinal bone mineral density decreased 1.2 percent.

One researcher conducted a randomized, double-blind study on the combination of IP and low-dose ERT.[62] Eighty-three post-menopausal women participated in this year-long multicenter study. Twenty-four women took a double placebo, thirty-one took a placebo plus conjugated estrogens in a dose of 0.3 mg per day, and twenty-eight women took the same dose of conjugated estrogens plus 200 mg of IP three times a day.

> There is some evidence that ipriflavone may be helpful as an adjunct to estrogen in maintaining bone density, but studies are inconsistent.

The placebo group showed a decrease in forearm bone density measured by DPA at one year, the conjugated estrogren group had an average bone loss of 1.4 percent, and the conjugated estrogen and IP group experienced increased BMD (+5.6%). The difference was significant.

Another one-year study randomized 105 Caucasian early postmenopausal women into five groups: a control group taking 500 mg of calcium; a low-dose HRT group (25 mcg/day 17 ß-estradiol estrogen patch plus the progestin medrogestone 5 mg/day for 12 days/month); a high-dose HRT group (50 mcg/day transdermal 17 ß-estradiol plus medrogestone 5 mg/day for 12 days/month); an ipriflavone group taking 600 mg a day;

and an ipriflavone combined with low-dose HRT group.[63] All were on a diet of 1,490 calories a day, including 73 grams of protein, 50 grams of lipids, 187 grams of carbohydrates, and 1550 mg of calcium.

Ninety-six women completed the study, with 81.8 percent observing the dietary regimen. Compared with baseline, the only significant change in vertebral bone mineral density measured by DPA was in the control group, in which vertebral bone mineral density decreased 3.41 percent. Mean BMD in the high-dose HRT group increased 1.84 percent, increased 0.11 percent in the ipriflavone group, and decreased 0.22 percent in the combined ipriflavone/HRT group. BMD was not significantly different in the low-dose HRT group where it decreased 0.55 percent.

Another study randomized eighty postmenopausal women aged forty to forty-nine to 500 mg of calcium per day, 200 mg of ipriflavone three times daily, 0.3 mg of conjugated estrogen per day, or 400 mg of IP plus 0.3 mg of conjugated estrogen per day. All treatment groups also received 500 mg of calcium each day.

There was a high dropout rate, and only fifty-two women completed the trial. Compared with baseline, vertebral bone density measured by DXA decreased significantly in the control and low-dose conjugated estrogen groups and increased significantly in both IP groups at one and two years.[64] The difference between both ipriflavone groups and the other two groups was significant. Ipriflavone had no effect on the vaginal maturation index (a measure of estrogen effect), which predictably improved in both groups receiving the conjugated estrogens.

Ipriflavone Versus Calcitonin

Over a year's time, forty postmenopausal women with a BMD greater than two points below the mean for age-matched controls were studied in a controlled but not blinded study comparing salmon calcitonin with ipriflavone.[65] Both treatments significantly increased bone mineral density. The increase was 4.3 percent in the ipriflavone group and 1.9 percent in the calcitonin group (the between-group difference was significant). Four patients in the IP group experienced gastric pain. In the calcitonin group, one patient reported itching and another complained of nosebleeds.

Summary

There is little reliable evidence supporting the use of ipriflavone for reducing fractures. Ipriflavone alone is not an effective treatment for bone loss in women without ovaries. Combining ipriflavone with estrogen or vitamin D may reduce but does not eliminate bone loss. Although five of eight placebo-controlled trials showed that ipriflavone maintained BMD in vertebrae or wrists of menopausal women, the most recent and largest trial showed no benefit of ipriflavone in maintaining bone density or reducing vertebral fractures in postmenopausal women. Also, a type of white blood cell decreased in a significant number of women, which may indicate decreased immune system function and increased susceptibility to infections.

PART THREE

Will HRT Prevent Disease, Preserve Your Mind, and Keep You Young?

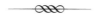

CHAPTER TEN

Hormone Therapy and Osteoporosis

If you want to prevent falls and fractures, there are better options than hormones.

The mother of one of us is seventy-three years old, weighs ninety-two pounds, has advanced Parkinson's disease, and falls every day. So far she has broken a toilet tank and bashed holes in the walls when she's fallen, but she hasn't broken any bones. Her forty-one-year-old son was the member of the family who slipped on the kitchen floor and broke his hip.

The point is that bones break. Osteoporosis may—or may not—have something to do with it.

As we discussed earlier, scaring women about their bone strength has become a burgeoning industry. Ads depict women slumped in wheel chairs and urge us to "talk to our doctors about osteoporosis" before it's too late. Free bone mineral density tests are offered to see "how much we've lost."

So what's the fuss? Shouldn't we talk to our doctors? Shouldn't we take care of ourselves? What's wrong with a free test?

What's wrong is that behind all this great national concern is an entire industry that stands to profit from turning a risk factor into a disease. And profit they do, as an entire generation of women is being encouraged to take hormones for many, many years.

Redefining Osteoporosis

We believe that osteoporosis is *not* a disease, but simply one risk factor for bone fracture; in the same way that high cholesterol is one risk factor for heart disease. Although preventing osteoporosis is one of the things we should be trying to do to prevent fractures, it is not—as the pharmaceutical industry would have us believe—the only thing.

> We believe that osteoporosis is *not* a disease, but simply one risk factor for bone fracture; in the same way that high cholesterol is one risk factor for heart disease.

Osteoporosis is a disease of fragile bones that leads to an increased risk of fracture. Fragile bones have less mass than normal bones; that is, a fragile bone weighs less than a normal bone of the same size. In addition, fragile bones have lost some of the microscopic structure that gives them strength.

Why Bones Break

Aside from the family genes that give some of us lighter bones, here is a list indicating what seems to put women at risk for bone fractures in old age:

- Lack of lean muscle mass, making us less strong and more likely to fall
- Use of long-acting tranquilizers, antidepressants, and other drugs that lead to dizziness and falls
- Inappropriate footwear that makes it more likely to fall
- Poor lighting, slippery rugs, and other hazards around the house
- Thinness
- Immobility or sedentary lifestyle
- Removal of ovaries, especially before natural menopause
- Low calcium intake
- Low levels of vitamin D intake
- High intakes of caffeine, alcohol, carbonated drinks, and high-protein foods
- Diets high in animal protein
- Cigarette smoking
- Alcoholism
- Untreated hyperthyroidism or hyperparathyroidism, both of which can cause bone loss
- Long-term use of oral steroid therapy or anticonvulsants
- Extreme physical exertion in premenopausal women (Activities such as running marathons, professional ballet dancing, and Olympic-level gymnastics may stop menstrual cycles and lead to bone loss.)

The exact definition of osteoporosis, however, is controversial. In 1994, based on bone mineral density, the World Health Organization created the following categories:

- Normal: Bone mineral density within 1 standard deviation of the average for young adult women
- Osteopenia: Bone mineral density 1.0 to 2.5 standard deviations below the average for young adult women
- Osteoporosis: Bone mineral density greater than 2.5 standard deviations below the average for young adult women
- Severe osteoporosis: Bone mineral density greater than 2.5 standard deviations below the average for young adult women and one fragility fracture

An Epidemic of a Disease or a Diagnosis?

Using the World Health Organization's definition of osteoporosis, the most conservative estimate is that 20 percent of postmenopausal women have osteoporosis,[1] although some researchers estimate the number is closer to 50 percent.[2]

The claim by some that half of women with osteoporosis will eventually fracture a bone is misleading. Researchers who made this prediction arrived at their conclusion by adding together the rate of wrist, hip, and vertebral fractures of the women they studied and dividing by the number of women in the study.[3] Some women included had multiple fractures. Calculating this way, one

The Truth About Hip Fractures

The chance of death from hip fracture has been used in the marketing of products to prevent, treat, or identify osteoporosis. These fractures, however, may not cause as many health problems as women have been led to believe.

Hip fracture rates are higher for women over the age of eighty. As osteoporosis researcher Steven R. Cummings at the University of California Medical Center in San Francisco writes, "Hip fractures may often be a marker and not the cause of declining health and impending death. Most patients who suffer a hip fracture have severe concomitant illness that accounts for much of the increased mortality after hip fracture."[4]

Interestingly, even though white women are most likely to have hip fractures, they are the least likely to die afterward. In a study of 712,027 persons covered by Medicare, white women experienced the lowest mortality rate following a fracture of the hip—17.2 per 1,000 person months, compared with 22.9 for black women, 33.5 for black men, and 33.7 for white men.[5] This has important public health implications, which drug manufacturers looking for the most profitable market may ignore. Although hip fractures and fear of hip fractures may be most common among white women, the lethality of hip fractures may be much worse for other populations.

woman with four fractures counts as four women, quadrupling the actual risk.

Not only is the arithmetic misleading, but also the researchers aren't taking into account the fact that wrist, hip, and vertebral fractures are all very different and have different health implications.

A hip fracture, especially in the frail elderly, may put a woman in bed for an extended period of time, increasing her chances of pneumonia, pulmonary embolism, and death. Vertebral fractures may or may not be painful and are rarely life-threatening. A wrist fracture does not compromise mobility.

So, is osteoporosis an epidemic of a disease? Or is it more accurately an epidemic of a diagnosis?

The Truth About Osteopenia

Osteopenia is even weaker at predicting individual risk of fracture. Its main use seems to be as a label to convince women they need hormone replacement therapy or other drug treatment to prevent "progression" to osteoporosis.

Not only may osteopenia not progress to osteoporosis, but osteopenia may also not even reflect bone loss. Bruce Ettinger, M.D., director of research for the Kaiser Permanente Medical Care Program in San Francisco, notes that a bone mineral density test done on a woman who is fifty-five may meet the definition of osteopenia *even if she has exactly the same BMD she had when she was twenty-five!*[6]

According to Dr. Ettinger, "If someone is 5 [foot] 3 at menopause and has been since adolescence, we don't say she's lost height." He goes on to say that osteopenia is "a real scary word [that] gets attached to something that may not be bone loss at all."[7]

In addition to instigating unnecessary "treatment," the diagnosis of osteopenia can have destructive effects. Sherry, a fifty-one-year-old woman who lifts weights three times weekly at the gym, recently returned from a trip to the Sierras where she backpacked fifty pounds for fifty miles. Her family doctor did a test for BMD and told her she had osteopenia. Given her strength and agility, Sherry probably doesn't need to worry about breaking bones unless she falls off a cliff! Yet her self-image as a superwoman changed overnight. Now she thinks she is weak and vulnerable. Will this actually cause her to reduce her bone-strengthening exercise?

Calcium Makes Estrogen More Effective

High intake of calcium makes estrogen more effective.[8] Women who decide to take estrogen but want to take the lowest dose can maximize the effectiveness of low estrogen doses by high calcium intake.

More than a decade ago, when most researchers considered 0.625 mg conjugated estrogens per day necessary to prevent bone loss, Bruce Ettinger, M.D., predicted, "By simply augmenting calcium intake to 1500 mg per day, women may be adequately protected while taking half the usual dosage of estrogen."[9]

Conversely, Dr. Ettinger also stated that very low intake of calcium, perhaps less than 300 mg per day, may diminish or abolish estrogen's protection.

Yet when a health care provider handles osteopenia intelligently, the result can be completely different. At seventy, Elizabeth was extremely healthy and active. However, before she went abroad for several months, she wanted to talk to her physician about her BMD test, which had shown osteopenia.

Her physician asked her about other risk factors, including easily broken bones in family members. Elizabeth thought for a moment and then said that her eight-year-old granddaughter, a gymnast, had broken her arm falling off a balance beam. The woman and her doctor agreed *that* certainly wasn't a familial risk factor and that she probably had little to fear from osteopenia. Instead of taking hormones and thinking of herself as someone with a "disease," Elizabeth decided to start calcium supplementation, take up weightlifting, and continue with her travels.

Risk Factors for Fractures

Fractures are a major problem for older women in the United States and northern Europe. This condition is less a problem in women in other parts of the world, including Japan.[10]

What explains this discrepancy? While the exact contribution of each factor is not known, it is clear that race, ethnicity, body build, diet, smoking, and physical activity have tremendous impact on a woman's risk of fracture in old age.

White women are more likely to have osteoporosis-related fractures than are women of any other racial or

What Works?

Osteoporosis itself is not the problem; fractures are what lead to disability and death in old age. According to the NIH Consensus Conference report, the evidence for fracture prevention is as follows:

- Calcium supplements increase spine bone mineral density and reduce vertebral and nonvertebral fractures. Vitamin D supplements reduce hip and other nonvertebral fractures.

- Bisphosphonates (alendronate, etidronate, risedronate) increase bone mineral density at the spine and hip and reduce the risk of vertebral fractures. Alendronate and risedronate reduce the risk of subsequent nonvertebral fractures.

- HRT decreases the risk of vertebral and nonvertebral fractures. Observational studies show reduced risk of hip fracture, but the HERS trial indicated no reduction in hip fracture after four years.

- Salmon calcitonin has positive effects on bone mineral density at the spine, but there is not yet any strong evidence regarding its effect on fracture risk.

- Raloxifene has been shown to reduce the risk of vertebral fracture but not hip fracture.

- Fall prevention and the use of hip protector garments "have been promising."

ethnic group.[11] Lifetime risk of hip fracture is approximately 16 percent for white women aged fifty, but only 6 percent for African American women.[12]

Within each group, women who are slender are more likely to fracture than heavier women.[13] Obesity protects against osteoporosis.[14] Women who are physically active have denser bones and fewer fractures in old age.

White women are more likely to have osteoporosis-related fractures than are women of any other racial or ethnic group.

Some medical conditions also increase the risk of fracture. These include kidney disease, liver disease, hypercortisolism, hyperthyroidism, hyperparathyroidism, and gastrectomy.

What Women Hear About Their Risk

None of this is what women usually hear. They hear that osteoporosis is caused by menopause.

Women are constantly warned that half of all fifty-year-old women will eventually experience a fracture. They are told that menopausal women need bone density screenings to determine whether they are at high risk. They have been indoctrinated to believe that all women, especially women with low bone mass, should start hormone therapy during or even before menopause.

These messages are misleading. We disagree with the almost universal message that nearly all women should use hormone therapy for bone health. We believe that nonhormonal drugs to prevent fractures are over-promoted as well. The claim that bone density screening during menopause accurately predicts risk of individual fracture is exaggerated.

BMD Screenings Encourage Medicalization of Menopause

Many people assume that osteoporosis screening must be a "good" thing. They don't recognize its limitations or how it plays into the medicalization of menopause. The importance of bone density screening appears in most osteoporosis materials, so it is no wonder that many menopausal women feel that baseline or regular bone density measurements should be part of their health care.

At the 2000 National Institute of Health's consensus conference on osteoporosis, however, virtually every speaker who talked about BMD screening questioned its value by noting that it is not a good predictor of fracture. The National Women's Health Network is concerned that bone density screening, either intentionally or coincidently, hooks women into a system in which drug prescriptions are their most likely choice. It is not a coincidence that much of the information on the dangers of osteoporosis and the value of bone screening and actual bone screening equipment all are paid for by pharmaceutical companies making osteoporosis products. (See "A Case Study: The Merck Launch of Fosamax" on pages 168–169.)

The Network is also concerned about the dissemination of misinformation about bone density. We do not recommend routine bone density screening for women younger than sixty-five. However, women who are at "high risk" for osteoporosis, because of early removal of ovaries or long-term steroid use, may decide to use screening earlier to learn if their bone mass is unusually low compared with women of their age.

Several techniques are currently available or are being developed to measure bone density. They vary in availability, cost, accuracy, reproducibility, and what they actually measure. While bone densitometry can show loss of bone mass, screening cannot predict how rapidly someone will lose bone and, most important, cannot predict whether someone will actually have fractures. Bone loss is neither constant nor predictable. Knowing someone's bone mass does not predict how fast that woman will lose bone in the future: A woman with low bone mass may end up losing at a very slow rate, and a woman with much higher bone mass may end up losing rapidly. Some instruments used to measure bone mass have a 1 or 2 percent margin of error, which may be similar to the amount of bone loss for some women between annual or biannual screenings. The loss could either be missed or exaggerated because the test lacks precision. Bone mass in postmenopausal women has been shown to demonstrate seasonal variations, so differences between two BMD readings could reflect this.[15] Furthermore, any time a woman hears that she has "low" bone mass, she must ask whether her bones are being compared with women her own age or with younger women at peak bone mass.

The entire field of bone density measurement is changing so rapidly that many perimenopausal women may want to wait a decade, when skeletal health measurements may be better predictors. No study has shown that measurements taken at age fifty accurately predict later fractures.[16] Studies have shown, however, that bone density measurements in women at sixty-five have some predictive value.[17] In the enthusiasm for osteoporosis screening, many health practitioners now recommend a "baseline" screening for perimenopausal or menopausal age women, but speakers at a recent osteoporosis conference noted that the pace of technological change in the bone density field is so rapid that women are being screened at age fifty with technology that will be obsolete by the time they have a second screening at age sixty-five.[18] There are also new urine and blood tests that measure how much active bone loss is occurring (however, at this time there is too much variability in these tests to rely on them).

A meta-analysis of eleven prospective cohort studies published between 1985 and 1994, with about 90,000 person years of observation time and more than 2,000 fractures, concluded, "There is a wide overlap in the bone densities of patients who develop a fracture and those who do not. Thus, bone mineral density can identify people who are at an increased risk of developing a fracture, but it cannot with any certainty identify individuals who will develop a future fracture."[19]

For a comprehensive review of the literature on bone density issues, the Network highly recommends the excellent "Bone Mineral Density Testing: Does the Evidence Support Its Selective Use in Well Women?" published by the British Columbia Office of Health

Bone Mineral Density Screening: Help or Hindrance?

Ads and company-sponsored educational materials intentionally blur the line between preventing bone loss and preventing fracture—which are two very different things, even though the FDA accepts prevention of bone loss as evidence for anti-fracture efficacy by estrogens and estrogenlike products.[20] There is no linear relationship between bone density and fracture risk. While women with the thickest bones have fewer fractures than women with the thinnest bones, the significance of bone loss is not so clear for women in the middle range.

At a consensus conference of the world's osteoporosis experts, convened by the National Institutes of Health in 2000, several leading researchers agreed that studies have failed to prove that a bone density measurement taken at menopause predicts likelihood of fracture.

The NIH consensus panel stopped short of direct criticism of the use of BMD testing for predicting fractures. It did, however, raise concerns about the accuracy of BMD testing and the difficulty in establishing useful standards for comparability between different devices. Panel members recommended that more comprehensive ways of assessing risk for fracture should be studied. According to the draft report issued by the expert panel,

> It has been suggested that the diagnosis of osteoporosis should depend on risk-based assessment. . . . Consideration of risk factors in conjunction with BMD will likely improve the ability to predict fracture risk. This approach needs to be tested in appropriate prospective studies.[21]

Technology Assessment.[22] We agree with the conclusions of this very comprehensive review:

> Research evidence does not support either whole populations or selective bone mineral density testing of well women at or near menopause as a means to predict future fractures. On some issues, evidence is insufficient because the research has not been done. Existing research evidence, though imperfect, indicates substantial limitations of BMD testing.

The greatest concern is that the BMD measurement will misdirect treatment efforts away from the majority of women who will ultimately suffer fractures by focusing attention on the minority who have low bone density. In addition, BMD testing will focus attention on bone mineral density, which is only one of the many risk factors, the alteration of which may or may not lead to fracture reduction.

The Impact of ERT/HRT on Bone Loss and Fractures

It is true that standard doses of ERT can slow normal bone loss in most women and can reduce the risk of hip fractures during the time it is taken and for several years afterward.[23]

Several studies have shown similar delay of bone loss and a reduced fracture rate in women taking HRT.[24, 25, 26, 27, 28, 29, 30] Articles also refer to estrogen increasing bone density by up to 5 percent,[31, 32] but approximately

15 percent of women given estrogen continue to lose bone.[33] Also, as we have noted, increased bone density does not necessarily mean that bones are stronger.

It will be the year 2007 before the Women's Health Initiative will be able to answer questions about the benefits and safety issues related to estrogen and HRT in the prevention of fractures. Nevertheless, it is now routine for health practitioners to encourage women at menopause (and increasingly before menopause) to begin long-term hormone use for the prevention of osteoporosis.

The emphasis on taking hormones at perimenopause or menopause is based on the thinking that the most rapid bone loss takes place during the first six years after menstruation ceases. Therefore, this thinking goes, hormonal "treatment" has the greatest impact on reducing bone loss if begun within three years after the onset of menopause.[34]

Recent studies show that this concept is only partially true and that the importance of preventing early bone loss at menopause seems to have been overemphasized. Longitudinal studies have shown that bone loss continues or even accelerates with increasing age.[35] According to Dennis Black, Ph.D., of the University of California San Francisco, "It is becoming clear that, at least at sites other than the spine, bone loss continues unabated into the oldest age ranges and probably accelerates at the hip, the most important region for predicting hip fractures."[36]

Even people who promote hormones for osteoporosis prevention debate whether women should start taking hormones before or after menopause. Because bone loss similar to the normal loss during menopausal years sets in as soon as hormones are stopped, estrogen started at menopause, even if taken for as long as ten years, does not protect women into their late seventies. Serious fractures are most common in the elderly, the average age of hip fracture being eighty.[37, 38]

As a result, treatment might have to be life long, possibly thirty or more years, with all the associated risks of long-term ERT/HRT use.[39] This knowledge has led experts to question the idea that hormone treatment for osteoporosis prevention beginning before or at menopause is worthwhile or cost-effective.

Starting estrogen before menopause may also increase breast cancer risks without increasing osteoporosis benefits. A meta-analysis of observational studies on estrogen replacement therapy found that studies in which estrogen therapy was started before menopause showed a much greater increase in breast cancer than did studies of women who started estrogen after menopause.[40]

A woman can make her decision about hormones for osteoporosis prevention many years after menopause. The emphasis on menopause as a time for intervention has more to do with it being an easily identifiable marker in a woman's life than with it being the optimal time for intervention. It may also have to do with the fact that women are still working at that age and are more likely to have health insurance that covers prescription drugs than are elderly women. The Rancho Bernardo Study of 740

> A woman can make her decision about hormones for osteoporosis prevention many years after menopause.

women over sixty who had chosen to take hormones found that there was no significant difference in bone mineral density between women who started estrogen at menopause and those who started after age sixty. The former group had twenty years of follow-up, and the latter group had nine years.[41]

Even the researchers for the Osteoporotic Fracture Research Group (a prospective study of 9,704 non-black women, sixty-five years or older), while emphasizing their view that estrogen is most effective if initiated soon after menopause and continued indefinitely, concluded that *current* use of estrogen in women of that age, whether started "early" (up to five years after menopause) or "late" (more than five years after menopause), reduces the risk for fractures.

Similarly, with hip fracture reduction, the Swedish Hip Fracture Study Group (which compared 1,327 women aged fifty to eighty-one with hip fractures to 3,262 randomly selected controls without hip fractures) identified that present or recent use of estrogen or hormone therapy was required for optimum fracture reduction. Long-term use of hormones seemed to benefit women who were still taking hormones or who had only stopped taking them within the past five years. Five years after stopping, no significant reduction in risk remained. This study also showed that a woman doesn't need to start hormones at menopause to reduce hip fractures. The authors concluded, "Once duration of use was taken into account we found similar protective effects of treatment whenever it was initiated in relation to the time of menopause."[42]

Dennis Black has argued that

[S]topping bone loss at age sixty-five to seventy can still prevent most instances of very low bone mass in women over eighty, that screening at age sixty-five can more precisely identify risk of hip fracture at age eighty, and that treatment beginning at age sixty-five may be more cost-effective than earlier screening and treatment.[43]

Smaller doses of estrogen may be just as effective as the usual doses in preventing fractures. The FDA has approved conjugated estrogens for osteoporosis at a dose of 0.625 mg per day. Similar doses of other types of estrogens are also approved to prevent bone loss. A few studies have found equally good bone density results with a half-strength dose of estrogen combined with calcium supplements.[44, 45, 46]

In 1998, the FDA approved the 0.3 mg estrogen pill Estratab as adequate protection against osteoporosis based on a two-year study of 406 women sponsored by Solvay Pharmaceuticals, Estratab's manufacturer.[47] The study compared the 0.3 level of estrogen with 0.625 or 1.25 levels of estrogen or with a placebo and found that all three levels of estrogen produced significant increases in bone mineral density of the lumbar spine, total hip, and whole body, compared with baseline and placebo.

Though bone mineral density was greater in the highest estrogen group, the authors concluded, "The results of this study indicate that doses of esterified estrogen as low as 0.3 mg per day, when combined with the daily supplementation of 1,000 mg of calcium, are

Is Osteoporosis Just a Women's Problem?

Maybe not. Most osteoporosis research has assumed that differences in fracture rates between men and women are due solely to menopause. Yet not all women lose significant bone mass during the transitional menopausal years, and both women and men lose bone density steadily as they age.

There are many other differences between men and women that affect bone strength and likelihood of fracture, especially in industrialized nations. For one thing, men develop larger and denser bones as young adults than do women. For another, women are encouraged to be thin throughout their lives. And, until relatively recently, women were actively discouraged from being strong or athletic. They're far more sedentary than men.

There's also a numbers bias. Since there are twice as many women as men over age seventy-five in the United States, there are always going to be more women than men with any age-related condition—including osteoporosis.

effective in preventing postmenopausal bone loss as evidenced by spine, hip, and whole body BMD changes."[48]

The 0.3 mg dose showed the desired positive effect on bones without the unwanted problem of endometrial changes. However, endometrial changes take at least a year, so this study wasn't long enough to be reassuring. A progestin should still be used even with low-dose estrogen regimens. A Swedish study found that ultra-low doses (7.5 mcg of 17-ß-estradiol per twenty-four hours) delivered by vaginal rings for the treatment of vaginal dryness also prevented bone loss in women over sixty.[49]

In a study that may help explain why low dosages of estrogen seem to be protective, the Osteoporotic Fracture Research Group found that one out of four women aged sixty-five and older who had undetectable levels of estrogen in their blood had increased risk of hip and vertebral fractures, independent of bone mineral density. They concluded,

> This association suggests that the risk of fractures in these women could be substantially reduced even with low-dose estrogen replacement therapy. . . . There is [also] a dose-response relation between serum estradiol concentration and the risk of breast cancer. Thus, maintaining low, but detectable, serum estrogen concentrations might reduce the risk of fracture without increasing the risk of breast and endometrial cancer.[50]

Although this is conjectural, it is interesting. It led the *New England Journal of Medicine* to run an editorial stating, "The evidence, then, suggests that the current recommended estrogen doses, particularly for women over sixty-five years of age, may be higher than required to maintain skeletal health. Lower doses are more likely to be acceptable to women because they cause fewer side effects."[51] Keep in mind that although low-dosage estrogen is increasingly accepted as a way to maintain bone density, the lower dose has not yet been proven to reduce fractures.[52]

Estrogen patches have been approved for use in prevention of osteoporosis. Theoretically, the patch should cause fewer effects on the liver and gallbladder than oral estrogen, but there is no data on this yet.

New Drugs to Prevent Bone Loss and Fractures

Calcitonin, a hormone produced by the parathyroid glands that helps control calcium levels in the body, is approved for the treatment of osteoporosis.

Until recently, calcitonin was only available in the United States as a fairly expensive injection. Its side effects are loss of appetite, nausea, diarrhea, and flushing of the face and hands.[53] It is somewhat effective in preventing bone loss and reducing fractures.[54] Salmon calcitonin is now available in a more convenient form as the nasal spray Miacalcin. The spray has fewer side effects than the injection (except for people with a rare allergic reaction to salmon).

Although there have been encouraging reports about modest but not significant increases in spine bone density and reduction in spine fracture occurrence, the value of this product to prevent loss of bone density and reduce hip fractures needs to be studied further.[55] Because calcitonin has a pain-relieving effect, it may be particularly beneficial for spinal fractures that are causing pain.[56]

The Medical Letter compared Miacalcin with another new osteoporosis treatment product, Fosamax, and concluded, "Miacalcin offers the least concern about safety, but its effectiveness is limited. Fosamax is probably more effective, but its long-term safety remains to be established."[57] Miacalcin is the most expensive method of osteoporosis prevention or treatment on the market, so cost will be a major barrier for many women.[58]

Fosamax: A Complicated Regimen

Fosamax (alendronate) is a bisphosphonate approved in the United States for osteoporosis prevention. It has been shown to increase bone density and prevent fractures.[59, 60, 61, 62] It is proving to be more useful for treating osteoporosis than for preventing it.[63] It is most effective for reducing fractures in postmenopausal women who have "advanced" osteoporosis such as very low bone mineral density and/or multiple vertebral fractures.[64, 65] The anti-fracture benefit in women with low bone mass but without prevalent fractures is less.[66]

Fosamax researchers themselves suggest "targeted treatment of high-risk individuals (women with advanced osteoporosis) may be an effective means to prevent the greatest number of fractures while minimizing the economic costs and potential risks of therapy."[67] They suggest it would take more than four years of Fosamax treatment to see a significant reduction in fractures in women who do not have osteoporosis, but there are no studies of the effectiveness or safety of Fosamax when used for more than four years.[68]

For someone who wants to take a drug to prevent or treat osteoporosis, Fosamax is a possible alternative to

A Case Study: The Merck Launch of Fosamax

When a company launches a new product, it is like a war, with attacks on all fronts. Merck's campaign to promote Fosamax was no different.

In 1995, Merck submitted Fosamax to the FDA for approval. Ads to health care providers started soon after. Merck, however, was planning ahead and realized that many women weren't worrying about osteoporosis. Therefore, as one part of its comprehensive campaign, Merck gave a large grant to a leading consumer group for older women, with the explicit understanding that the group would use the grant to "educate" women to worry about osteoporosis. Merck obviously hoped this investment would raise the level of women's concern about the strength of their bones. To reinforce women's concern, Merck began running direct-to-consumer ads that featured frail older women in pain contrasted with vivacious, active seniors in control of their lives. The text implied that medication made the difference.

Next Merck took this newly created fear and concern and translated it into action. They began marketing bone density testing, first by making it more available, then by making it more affordable.[69] Even before Fosamax received FDA approval, Merck purchased a small company that

HRT. While the drug is still relatively new and therefore lacks a long-term safety record, it does not appear to have the blood clot and cancer risks that estrogen does.

In its first years on the market, Fosamax has given rise to a great number of reports of adverse drug reactions against it.[70] The FDA Regulatory Review Office manufactured bone density testing equipment and expanded its production to make more bone density machines.[71]

Merck also gave the National Osteoporosis Foundation a large grant to promote a toll-free number through which consumers, now having been "educated," could find the location of a nearby bone density screening center.[72] Because bone density screening isn't cheap, Merck added a final piece to its campaign: a public policy initiative to persuade the federal government to pay for bone density screening tests through Medicare. Merck also targeted private insurers at the state level with slick educational materials and drew up model legislation for distribution to state legislators, who could then argue for state funding so women could get free or inexpensive bone scans.

Having successfully persuaded women to worry about the strength of their bones and to have their bone density measured, Merck had created the perfect environment to sell its product. Every component of its campaign contributed to sales of Fosamax, the only nonhormonal drug approved at the time for osteoporosis prevention. The vast majority of women affected by Merck's effort don't know the true motivation behind the information they receive—much less who paid for it.

had to contact Merck, the manufacturer, more than once about misleading claims in violation of the Food, Drug and Cosmetic Act.[73] The original Fosamax regimen was complicated, and the large number of adverse reactions is thought to reflect the difficulty that patients had in complying with the instructions for safe use.

The four-year Fracture Intervention Trial Research Group's studies, supported by Merck, carefully instructed participants to take their Fosamax with at least four ounces of water in a fasting state and to not lie down or drink any other food or liquid for at least a half hour. Participants were also specifically told that calcium supplements, antacids, tetracycline, and other drugs could not be taken until after breakfast.

The researchers claim that if people followed the strict instructions, Fosamax did not significantly increase the risk of abdominal symptoms or gastrointestinal problems and that the risk of esophagitis was low and not significantly different from placebo.[74] However, abdominal pain, esophagitis, and damage to the mucosa of the upper gastrointestinal tract causing drug-induced ulcers are all side effects people have reported from Fosamax use.[75, 76, 77, 78]

In 2000, the FDA approved a new once-a-week regimen of Fosamax that puts the entire dose for one week into one pill. For osteoporosis prevention, the dose is 35 mg per week. For treatment of osteoporosis, it is 70 mg per week. This dose proved effective in reducing bone turnover and increasing bone density in a one-year trial. The weekly dose may be easier for women to take the drug without experiencing problems, since it reduces how often they must follow the complicated regimen. In the trial, safety and side effects appeared to be similar to those for the daily dose. It remains to be seen whether women using this higher dose outside of the strictly controlled environment of a clinical trial will experience increased adverse reactions.

Some of the restrictions on Fosamax use may be particularly difficult for people with osteoporosis to follow. Women must make sure they have a high calcium intake. Indeed, calcium supplements were given to women taking fewer than 1,000 mg per day in the Fracture Intervention Trial and to women in other bisphosphonate trials.[79] There is no evidence that bisphosphonates are effective without calcium. However, as the instructions from Merck say, it is extremely important that women not take calcium preparations at the same time as their Fosamax.[80] The woman who chooses to take Fosamax because she has a fracture may not be mobile. In one case, a bedridden woman took Fosamax with half a glass of water and developed large esophageal ulcers after seven days of treatment.[81] Because aspirin, other nonsteroidal anti-inflammatory drugs, and Fosamax all cause mucosal damage, it may not be appropriate to use both products at the same time.[82, 83]

In opposing FDA approval for Fosamax, the National Women's Health Network told the FDA Endocrinological and Metabolic Drugs Advisory Committee:

> We want to stress that we support the availability of nonhormonal treatments for osteoporosis, but at the same time we believe it is unwise to recommend their use for osteoporosis in a manner that exposes too many women to drug treatment. No side effect is worth it if a drug is not necessary in the first place.[84]

Other bisphosphonate drugs, including risedronate (Actonel), have entered the market, and the SERM raloxifene is heavily promoted for osteoporosis treatment. More drugs in these categories can be expected (see chapter 5).

Playing on Women's Fears

Now that osteoporosis is a "hot" topic, we see a flood of new products on the market promising the perfect prevention or treatment. We strongly support the availability of safe nonhormonal methods for osteoporosis treatment, but we want to caution you to be vigilant about claims of long-term efficacy or safety based on short-term studies.

We are particularly concerned about direct-to-consumer marketing that plays on women's fears of disabilities but does nothing to give them the information they need to make informed decisions about new products.

Hyping the dangers of osteoporosis serves a purpose for the pharmaceutical companies that sell hormones and other treatments. As new osteoporosis products reach the market, we want you to remember that most drugs have

Teach Girls to Build Bone

All women should be aware of the importance of building strong bones before age thirty-five and of developing health habits to maintain optimum bone strength after they reach "peak bone mass" in their thirties. Adolescent girls can increase bone mineral density by regularly participating in weight-bearing activity and consuming calcium.[85] The ability of bones to rebuild themselves diminishes with age.

only been researched for a relatively short time compared with the length of time women will need to take them to prevent fractures.

> Always keep in mind that exercise and nutrition can do more than drugs can to protect bones and provide other health benefits.

Women must evaluate whether to start long-term therapy with a product whose safety record is short-term. Always keep in mind that exercise and nutrition can do more than drugs to protect bones and also provide other health benefits. (See chapter 16, "Alternatives to Hormone Replacement Therapy.")

Bone Density Tests Used to Overcome Resistance to HRT

BMD measurements may be used to badger resistant women into using HRT. Statements such as, "Women who refuse HRT for osteoporosis prevention should be offered a BMD measurement,"[86] are worrisome, and there is increasing evidence that bone density screening does increase hormone use.

One randomized study of 140 menopausal women compared women who received a voucher for an immediate BMD measurement with women who received a voucher for a BMD measurement one year later. All women were offered hormone prescriptions. Sixty-four percent of the women who had immediate BMD testing filled their prescriptions, compared with only 20 percent of women who had not yet had BMD screenings.[87]

Another randomized trial of more than twelve hundred women aged forty-five to fifty-four mailed a follow-up questionnaire about hormone use and quality of life two years after the women had or had not had BMD screening. The researchers concluded, "Screening for low bone density significantly increases the use of HRT in this population but without any immediate adverse or positive effects on the quality of life." (Obviously a two-year follow-up study in this age group was not going to determine whether the hormones affected fracture rates.[88])

> Bone screening could be counterproductive if it results in less physical activity by exactly the women who need to strengthen bone mass!

Because bone density screening is often used to persuade women to take hormones, it is important that women recognize that many factors may cause bone loss. Before someone decides whether to take hormones based on BMD measurements, other possible causes of low bone density, including vitamin D deficiency and hyperparathyroidism, should be ruled out. The incidence of hyperparathyroidism is highest in postmenopausal women.[89]

A study that demonstrated that bone screening can be very influential in encouraging women to use estrogen replacement therapy showed that women who were told they had low BMD became fearful of falling and began to

Buyer Beware!

Before filling any prescription for drugs to prevent or treat osteoporosis, consider these points:

- The efficacy of all the drugs for osteoporosis prevention and treatment has been established in studies that test a combined regimen that includes calcium and vitamin D as well as the drug in question. We do not know whether these drugs work when women take them without calcium and vitamin D supplementation.[90] Most health care providers do not prescribe these supplements.
- There is a dearth of scientific evidence from clinical trials about osteoporosis and the benefits of drugs for women over age seventy-five. It is these women who are most at risk for hip fracture, but drugs have not been adequately tested for safety or efficacy in this age group.
- Most of the drugs for treatment and prevention of osteoporosis are too new to have a long-term record on safety or efficacy. ERT and HRT have the longest record, but these drugs are not risk-free.

limit their activities.[91] Bone screening could be counter-productive if it results in less physical activity by exactly the women who need to strengthen bone mass! The unintended, potentially fracture-increasing consequences of marketing bone density screening to women without giving them information to make health-promoting decisions need to be considered much more seriously.

High Bone Density and Cancer

There is one circumstance in which BMD may be helpful in decisions about taking hormones. The study done by the Osteoporotic Fractures Research Group has shown a strong association between high bone density and breast cancer:

> We have demonstrated that increased BMD of the radius, hip, or spine is significantly associated with an increased risk of subsequent breast cancer. . . . The association between BMD and breast cancer was similar in magnitude to the risk observed for other strong predictors of breast cancer.[92]

The association between high BMD and the risk of breast cancer is stronger in women with a family history of breast cancer than among women without this family history.[93] Thus, a high BMD reading may help women feel very good about a decision not to take hormones.

CHAPTER ELEVEN

Hormone Therapy and Heart Disease

HRT is unhealthy for some women, unproven for others.

Estrogen has never been proven to prevent heart disease in women. Nevertheless, hundreds of thousands of women may be taking ERT/HRT because a health care practitioner told them it would prevent heart disease.

This has been going on for some time, and despite mounting evidence that estrogen may actually cause heart attacks in some women, it doesn't seem to be changing.

Starting in 1998, solid evidence became available that shows ERT and HRT don't prevent further problems in women who already have heart disease. In 2000, early results from a large randomized trial reported that the first two years of hormones for healthy women didn't help at all. What's more, it seems that hormones may even hurt by actually causing heart attacks, blood clots, and strokes.

Despite these findings, women find themselves surrounded by messages saying estrogen prevents heart disease. Among these are direct-to-consumer ads and educational materials, which are available in health care providers' offices and clinics. Even some clinicians still say heart health is a reason to take hormones.

You will almost certainly experience this disconnect between the actual facts and what the rest of the world tells you. In this section, we attempt to list all the reasons why the medical community has been so positive about hormones and heart disease for so long and to explain the flaws in their reasoning.

Does Estrogen Make Women Healthy, or Do Healthy Women Take Estrogen?

One of the main reasons women are told to take estrogen is to prevent heart disease.[1, 2] We hear the consistent message from clinicians, news reports, magazines, and messages sponsored by drug companies that estrogen cuts heart disease in half.

What we are less likely to hear is the truth—that women who *choose* to take estrogen have only half as many heart attacks as women who don't.

What's the difference between these statements? Lots! Because women choose whether or not to take estrogen, there may be other differences between users and nonusers. For instance, estrogen users may have lower heart disease risk before they start using estrogen.

Studies of women undergoing natural menopause have found that those who later chose to take estrogen were less likely to get heart disease even *before* they began to take estrogen.[3, 4] The reason? Stud-
ies have found that ERT users are less likely to smoke and to have diabetes and are more physically active and leaner. One study even found estro-gen users had higher HDL cholesterol levels before they took estrogen. (HDL choles-terol, or high-density lipopro-tein, the "good" cholesterol, protects against the damage

> Studies of women undergoing natural menopause have found that those who later chose to take estrogen were less likely to get heart disease even *before* they began to take estrogen.

done by LDL cholesterol. LDL cholesterol, or low-density lipoprotein, is the bad kind that damages arteries.) Also, women who take ERT are more likely to make lifestyle changes that lower the risk of disease than are other women of the same social and economic group.[5, 6]

Moreover, health care providers may be less likely to prescribe estrogen to women who have higher risk of heart disease. Many women with a history of heart dis-ease or obvious risk factors for cardiovascular disease are told not to take estrogen because it can cause blood clots and worsen high blood pressure (these risks appear on the FDA label).[7] Studies that look at the likelihood of death in women on ERT/HRT can be skewed because women often stop using hormone preparations when they come down with a life-threatening illness such as

Give This to Your Health Care Provider!

Although data regarding heart disease and HRT are clear, your health care provider may still be under the "impression" that HRT may somehow be good for your heart. The following timeline will present the facts quickly.

1989   The first edition of *Taking Hormones and Women's Health*, published by NWHN, mentions a new trend among gynecologists to recommend ERT/HRT for heart disease prevention. *Taking Hormones* warns that this benefit of estrogen has not yet been proven.

1990   Wyeth-Ayerst, manufacturer of Premarin, asks the FDA to approve Premarin to prevent heart disease in women who have already had a hysterectomy. In public testimony, the Network opposes Wyeth's request by pointing out that every heart disease prevention drug used by men has been tested in a large randomized trial but that this has never been done for ERT/HRT.[8] Wyeth pays for many leading researchers to attend the meeting, and they argue that a large randomized trial of ERT/HRT isn't feasible. The FDA agrees with the Network and denies Wyeth's request.

1992   Bernadine Healy, M.D., in her first month as head of the NIH, tells Congress that she will ensure that the NIH study important women's health issues, including the effect of ERT/HRT on heart disease and cancer. The Network lobbies hard to make sure the trial starts. At various times, the trial is opposed by members of Congress, who think it is too expensive; by epidemiologists, who think the design is too complicated; and by leading gynecologists, who think the heart disease benefit is so well proven that it is unethical to ask women to accept the possibility that they might be randomized to a placebo. The Women's Health Initiative begins in 1993.

1993   Wyeth-Ayerst funds HERS to study women who already have heart disease. They not only hope that HRT will be beneficial for those women, but also that positive findings will supply more evidence that it prevents heart disease in healthy women and that FDA approval will follow.

1998   HERS results are announced: HRT does not help women who already have heart disease.[9] Proponents of estrogen argue that the trial was stopped too soon, that it used the wrong combination of estrogen and progestin, and that even if the results were accurate, they didn't apply to healthy women. This argument ignores the fact that the most widely used drug was tested and that there is no prevention drug known that helps healthy people but that is ineffective in those with the disease.

March 2000   The safety-monitoring committee of the Women's Health Initiative informs participants that women on ERT or HRT are more likely to have heart attacks, blood clots, or strokes than are women taking placebos.[10] The results receive some notice in mainstream media, but are not embraced by clinicians. Wolf Utian, M.D., executive director of the National American Menopause Society, tells the *New York Times* that these results "don't change my stance at all."[11]

June 2001   Women's Health Initiative researchers send participants another letter informing them that the increased risk of cardiovascular disease for women on hormones is still statistically significant after three years on the drug.

cancer.[12] All of these are fairly obvious reasons why the "fact" that estrogen users are less likely to have heart disease does not necessarily mean that estrogen prevents heart disease.

A Subtle Bias

Another, more subtle type of bias may be falsely inflating the apparent effectiveness of estrogen. A thought-provoking argument has been raised by Diana Petitti, an epidemiologist with the Kaiser Research Foundation, and others questioning whether the willingness of healthy people to take a pill every day in hopes of preventing chronic disease could be an indication that the person is also making other lifestyle choices that result in disease prevention.[13]

It's interesting that two studies found that volunteers who were very consistent about taking their assigned pill every day—even if it was a placebo!—were less likely to develop heart disease than volunteers who took their pills inconsistently.[14, 15] Since the placebo contained no active drug, researchers reason that the person's consistency in taking the pills probably indicated other health-promoting behavior. (Perhaps this group was also conscientious about exercising regularly and avoiding cheeseburgers.)

The researchers looked at over a dozen measurable factors known to influence heart disease and found the two groups apparently similar in every measurable way. This raises the important question of whether estrogen use merely identifies women who practice successful prevention behavior, rather than being a successful preventive intervention itself.

New Research: Should Healthy Women Take Estrogen?

What's really important is whether estrogen use changes the risk of heart disease in an individual woman. Unfortunately, the evidence can't tell us that yet. The best way to find the answer to that question would be to have many women volunteer to take either estrogen or a placebo and not tell them who was taking the real drug. After several years, we would discover if the women who took estrogen had fewer heart attacks than the women taking the placebo pills.

> What's really important is whether estrogen use changes the risk of heart disease in an individual woman. Unfortunately, the evidence can't tell us that yet.

Because heart disease does not usually occur in women until their sixties, this type of study would take a very long time to do. It's also expensive. So far, no drug company has been willing to fund such a study.

In the meantime, activist and political pressure has persuaded the federal government to begin the Women's Health Initiative. This study began in 1993 and will answer questions about the role of estrogen and HRT in women's health. Final results won't be available until most of the volunteers have been taking hormones for seven to nine years. However, early results were so dismaying that the researchers felt duty-bound to inform volunteers that, in contrast to the hope that ERT/HRT would reduce the risk of heart disease, during the first two years it actually *caused* more heart attacks and strokes.[16] This doesn't prove that ERT/HRT causes heart disease, and the trial is continuing so that a conclusive answer can be found. It does seem to argue against the common practice of health care providers to prescribe ERT/HRT for heart disease on the basis of observational studies.

What About Women Who Already Have Heart Disease?

Evidence about the effects of estrogen on women who already have heart disease is more conclusive, and the news isn't good.

Two large studies of women with heart disease have reported their results in the past two years. Both have found that ERT and HRT do not stop heart disease from progressing.

Nearly three thousand women with heart disease volunteered to be randomized to either an estrogen/progestogen combination pill or a placebo in the Heart and Estrogen/Progestin Replacement study (HERS).[17] They were monitored for over four years.

Even though their cholesterol levels improved, the women taking hormones were just as likely to have a heart attack or die from heart disease. In addition, the complications found in observational studies were seen again, strengthening the proof that HRT causes blood clots and gallbladder problems.

These findings were so clear that the researchers recommended that women with preexisting cardiovascular disease should not begin using HRT. Their recommendation was later reinforced when the American Heart Association issued a science advisory recommending that women with heart disease should not begin HRT.

What's more, the findings from this large trial were reinforced in the year 2000 by a smaller trial studying narrowing of the arteries (atherosclerosis). It reported that neither estrogen alone nor estrogen plus progestin stopped arteries from narrowing in women who had already been diagnosed with atherosclerosis before starting the study.[18] ERT and HRT didn't lower the risk of heart attack or other heart disease in these women. Just as in the HERS study, this failure to stop disease progression happened even though both ERT and HRT improved cholesterol levels.

The Bottom Line

These results also have important implications for the interpretation of further research on heart disease.

Because both HERS and other significant studies have found no benefit of estrogen on heart disease, in spite of beneficial effects on cholesterol, some researchers now argue that the cholesterol effects of estrogen are not relevant to heart disease effects. In other words, research that shows estrogen improves cholesterol levels should not be interpreted as having any implication for estrogen's effect on heart disease.

Clearly, women with heart disease shouldn't begin using HRT unless they have another reason to take it.

What about healthy women who are offered ERT or HRT to prevent heart disease? It is true that nearly every observational study that examines the experience of healthy women who are currently taking estrogen has found that heart disease rates are significantly lower, usually around 35 percent less.[19, 20, 21] Although not every study finds this benefit,[22] some researchers believe the positive findings are reinforced by other studies that look at the effect of estrogen on cholesterol levels and other risk factors for heart disease. Animal studies also show a benefit.[23]

> Research that shows estrogen improves cholesterol levels should not be interpreted as having any implication for estrogen's effect on heart disease.

In spite of these epidemiologic and animal findings, we believe that this type of evidence is insufficient to conclude that a drug is effective—especially a drug intended to be used for many years by healthy people.

Here's why: Drugs used in the primary prevention of heart disease in men are always tested in large and lengthy, randomized, double-blind trials. Until recently, this type of trial has not been done on women. Interestingly, the pooled results of all controlled trials to date, almost all of them short-term, found that healthy women assigned to ERT/HRT were *more* likely to experience cardiovascular problems than women who were given placebo pills.[24] A large, long-term randomized trial of ERT is especially important because observational trials that do not assign the estrogen to specific women may be biased in significant ways.

> It is always important to wait for the final results of randomized trials before advising healthy women to take hormones or other drugs with known health risks.

The surprising negative results of the HERS and atherosclerosis trials should serve as a clear warning. It is always important to wait for the final results of randomized trials before advising healthy women to take hormones or other drugs with known health risks.

Progestins: A Wild Card in the Deck

Since the late 1970s, women have been advised to add progestins to estrogen treatment to reduce the risk of endometrial cancer caused by estrogen alone. (This is the only reason to add progestins, so women who have had a hysterectomy use estrogen alone.)

By 1992, about one-third of all women taking estrogen also took progestins.[25] Yet estrogens and progestins often have opposite effects, and progestins can undo estrogen's beneficial effects on cholesterol levels. Some researchers even speculate that the HERS trial might have found a beneficial effect if women without a uterus had taken estrogen alone rather than estrogen plus progestin.

In the mid-1990s, the first substantial evidence emerged about the experience of women who take HRT.[26] Grodstein and others involved in the Nurses Health Study reported that women on HRT have a significantly lower rate of heart disease, similar to the nurses who take estrogen alone.[27] The results of this large observational study appear to confirm results from smaller studies of women who have chosen to use hormones, as well as short-term randomized trials that have looked at risk factors for heart disease.

The PEPI study, however, found differences among different types of progestins.[28] (The PEPI study is discussed in detail in chapter 14.) It found that all forms of HRT increased triglyceride levels, a possible risk factor for heart disease in women. Medroxyprogesterone, the most commonly used progestin, significantly interfered with the positive effect that estrogen alone has on HDL cholesterol levels. In contrast, however, micronized progesterone apparently had little effect on the beneficial cholesterol changes induced by estrogen.

Although these studies are encouraging, smaller studies combined with experimental work in animals raise some troubling questions about the safety of Provera when used as part of HRT.

These studies show that adding medroxyprogesterone in monkeys taking estrogen makes them less able to survive an induced heart attack.[29] A very small trial in women similarly showed that adding medroxyprogesterone to ERT reduced blood flow to the heart.[30]

Though not definitive, these small studies serve to remind us that studies that rely solely on risk factors or that simply observe the health of women who choose to use hormones don't necessarily predict the effects of a drug in preventing heart attacks and strokes.

Heart Disease: The Big Picture

Heart disease has been declining in the United States for the past thirty years. Heart disease rates in women peaked in 1962 and 1963 and since then have declined between 50 and 60 percent.[31]

The medicalization of menopause and the attempt to define postmenopausal life as a state of estrogen deficiency has provided the context for a skewed view of heart disease as a newly urgent problem for women, best treated by estrogen.[32]

Kathleen MacPherson, a nurse who conducts research on aging issues, has encouraged health activists to reexamine cardiovascular problems as diseases associated with aging, not hormone deficiency.[33] Others, including the authors of *The New Ourselves, Growing Older,* resist the concept that aging, *per se*, leads to any disease, since not all aging people develop these diseases.[34]

> If women are going to take an unproven pill to prevent heart disease, why not take something that does not cause cancer, costs less than estrogen, and in the case of aspirin has been shown to be effective in men?

In addition, much is known about the cause, prevention, and treatment of heart disease. Eating habits, exercise, and smoking (including exposure to secondhand smoke) all contribute to heart disease. These are all factors that women can alter on their own.

Meir Stampfer, a Harvard researcher involved in the Nurses Health Study testified at an FDA hearing on estrogen and heart disease, saying, "If we applied current knowledge, I believe we could reduce heart disease by 90 percent without estrogen."[35]

Low-dose aspirin, increased dietary intake of folate, and supplemental use of folic acid all have shown promise for preventing heart disease.

The effects of aspirin and folic acid have not been established by a randomized controlled trial in women. Yet if women are going to take an unproven pill to prevent heart disease, why not take something that does not cause cancer, costs less than estrogen, and—in the case of aspirin—has been shown to be effective in men?

Public health principles suggest that clinicians should use prevention interventions that are risk-free whenever possible. Given that so much is known about safe ways to lower women's risk of heart disease, it is disturbing that many clinicians are so enthusiastic about recommending hormone therapy to nearly all postmenopausal women.[36]

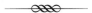

CHAPTER TWELVE

Does Hormone Therapy Preserve Mind, Mood, and Memory?

Although estrogen can boost the chemical function of brain cells in the lab, its effect on real people is another matter.

Women who are reluctant to take HRT may base the decision not to use hormones at least in part on the fact that there are other ways of lowering one's risk for osteoporosis and heart disease.

Nonhormonal alternatives to keep our brains sharp are not so clear. Guess who is making the most of this dilemma? The drug companies' latest big promotion is to convince us to use HRT to keep us from losing our minds. Because we associate problems of concentration and forgetfulness with age, and loss of mental capacity is terrifying for most of us, a "cure" via estrogen replacement therapy would greatly increase its marketability.

Alzheimer's disease, in particular, worries women because of its increasing prevalence, the duration of complete mental disability, and its social and financial costs to family members and to society.[1]

Estrogen's Effect on the Brain

Molecular biology studies indicate that estrogen can boost brain cells' chemical function, spur their growth, and protect them from toxins.[2, 3, 4] Barrett-Connor calls biological plausibility "estrogen's strongest suit."[5] Whether this basic science translates into estrogen actually functioning this way in human beings remains to be seen. One study used magnetic resonance imaging of the brain on postmenopausal women on estrogen as they completed memory tasks. The MRI detected increased brain activation patterns in the women being treated but saw no effect on actual performance of the tests.[6]

It is also not clear how estrogen's effect on the brain may be modified in combination with progestin. In the meantime, researchers working with monkeys have determined that the brain regularly makes new nerve cells (neurons) even in adults, which was previously thought not to happen.[7] If these results are confirmed in humans, women may feel there is hope for better brain function even without hormones.

Research that looks at the impact of ERT on memory and dementia (including Alzheimer's disease) has produced inconclusive and conflicting results. While several studies found ERT to be effective in maintaining cognitive function in Italian[8] and New York women[9, 10] and in lessening the risk of developing Alzheimer's disease among women from Minnesota,[11] others found that estrogen levels in the blood[12] or use of ERT/HRT[13, 14] were unrelated to cognitive function.

What Else Could It Be?

Women who note declines in memory should ask their health care providers about possible effects of medications they are taking, particularly interactions of multiple drugs. Also, mental exercise and stimulating experiences improve memory and keep function stable in the absence of stroke or falls that can inflict physiological damage on the brain.[15] There is also new evidence that physical exercise is good for maintaining memory.

Some researchers question the predominant view in western culture of inevitable physical and mental decline with age. Marian Cleeves Diamond, a neurophysiologist at the University of California Berkeley, dismisses claims about brain deterioration during aging as a myth.[16]

> One intriguing cross-cultural study of memory found no significant loss in short-term memory with age in China. The same study, conducted with subjects from the United States, showed people scoring progressively worse as they grew older.

For one thing, there is evidence of a strong social component to decreased mental acuity. The risk of Japanese American men developing Alzheimer's disease is nearly triple that of the risk for Japanese men in Japan,[17] and there is a significant excess of Alzheimer's cases in rural compared with urban areas of Quebec.[18] The disproportionate incidence of Alzheimer's disease among African Americans and Latinos,[19] the strong protective effect of education[20] even within racial groups,[21] social engagement,[22] emotional expression,[23] and linguistic capability[24] all suggest we should look at social and environmental explanations for brain deterioration as well as biological ones.[25, 26]

One intriguing cross-cultural study of memory found no significant loss in short-term memory with age in China, a culture that traditionally pays great respect to the elderly.[27] The same study, conducted with subjects from the United States where negative feelings about aging abound, showed people scoring progressively worse as they grew older.

This leads us to suspect that the best treatment to keep us mentally sound may be for all of us to improve our social attitudes, expectations, and practices toward elders.

Mood and Depression

Who wouldn't feel moody and depressed if described as a "pain-racked, petulant invalid" or a "castrate"—the language that Robert A. Wilson, M.D., used to describe his own mother in his best-selling book, *Feminine Forever.*[28]

Wilson's book influenced an entire generation of women and their health care providers. It is crammed with quotable gems that reflect his perspective that estrogen "deficiency" robs women of femininity and entrenches us in "menopausal negativism."[29]

Yet the widespread association of emotional trauma, moodiness, and depression with menopause is not well-supported by evidence. For many women, the onset of depression peaks during childbearing years and decreases after age forty-five. It does not increase during menopause.[30]

Furthermore, health interviews with 8,679 women and men, aged twenty-five to seventy-five, from doctors' practices in the Netherlands, showed no gender differences in changes in insomnia, tiredness, irritability, depression, headache, and other symptoms over time.[31]

Sonja and John McKinlay and colleagues have also studied a large sample of middle-aged and older women in Massachusetts for many years. They found that while women who were surgically menopausal had high depression rates, women anticipating and experiencing natural menopause did not and actually viewed menopause with nonchalance. Clearly, social factors were far more important in explaining depression.[32]

> For many women, the onset of depression peaks during childbearing years and decreases after age forty-five. It does not increase during menopause.

Why Studies of ERT and Brain Function Frequently Don't Make Sense

Studies of ERT and brain function in women contain many methodological problems that make it difficult to use this research for individual decision making. These include:

Selection Bias   Health care providers may be less likely to prescribe ERT as a prevention regimen to women who are ill or who have less cognitive capacity. Cognitively impaired women are more likely to forget to take their medication or to report that they are using it. Many studies do not adequately describe participants, making detection of selection bias difficult or impossible. Schneider et al. found that Alzheimer's patients eligible for clinical trials are not representative of the overall clinic population.[33]

Failure to Control Intervening Variables   Because ERT is relatively expensive and requires a visit to a health care provider for prescriptions, those who use it are more likely to be from higher income groups. In the United States, high income generally equates with more education and better health status. Women with more education score better on memory tests and are less likely to develop Alzheimer's disease, dementia, and memory loss than women with less education. Because the people most likely to use ERT are the least likely to develop cognitive dysfunction, observational studies that do not take this into account are ignoring an important explanation for their findings.

Confounding Improvement in Cognitive Performance with Relief from Physiologic Effects of Menopause
Estrogen relieves bothersome symptoms that some women experience in perimenopause—including hot flashes and attendant sleep disruption. Being rested enhances our ability to think and recall information, making the independent effects of estrogen on the brain more difficult to measure and analyze.

Heterogeneity in Treatments and in Tests of Outcome
Haskellet et al.[34] and Yaffe et al.[35] point out that the ability to systematically analyze research in this area suffers from lack of measures of cognitive impairment and standardization of treatment. The variety of formulations of ERT/HRT delivery, all evolving continuously, make it difficult to compare treatment effects, particularly over time. Similarly, researchers use a variety of tests to measure memory and cognitive function, including many that are not validated.

Small Sample Sizes and Short Duration of Studies
The ten controlled trials in Haskell and colleagues' comprehensive review had from 18 to 125 participants and followed the women from as little as six weeks to as long as three years.[36] On average, the trials had 43 participants, and average duration was eight months. Findings are always more valid with larger samples and a longer period of observation.

Proxy Respondents Underestimate Hormone Use
Most studies of Alzheimer's disease and hormone use rely on family members or caregivers to answer questions. In general, proxy respondents underreport use of medication. If a study relies on proxies for information about hormone use in Alzheimer's cases but on direct informants for its use in controls (as many studies do), the percentage of hormone users in Alzheimer's sufferers will be underestimated and the hormone use will be measured as protective.

Conflict of Interest   Industry-sponsored studies are more likely to show their product is effective than are independently funded studies. The affiliations and financial disclosures of participants in the Alzheimer's Consensus Conference show how deeply imbedded the pharmaceutical industry is in the creation of health policy in this area.[37] The conference itself was sponsored by three companies with financial interest in its conclusions.

Wilson, showing that he too is attuned to the role of social factors in a way that neatly matches his mysogyny, provides this analysis:

> It is on the next lower rung of the social scale that the most pitiful cases of menopausal negativism are usually found. In the vast social and spiritual wasteland below the comfortable suburban strata, in the drabness of the lower middle class, many factors combine to render a woman psychologically helpless. Typically, such a woman, shackled to a dull, common-place man, lacks that margin of imagination, cultural interest, and developed taste that helps upperclass women to fight back against menopausal despair, no matter how misguided their methods.[38]

Some women do report "moodiness," "irritability," and other mood-related symptoms during the years leading up to menopause, but there is no evidence that these symptoms are linked to hormone fluctuations.

Depression Neither Prevented Nor Treated by ERT

Studies of the prevention or treatment of depression using estrogen therapy are flawed by the same problems that plague cognitive function studies, and they report inconsistent results.[39] The most common error found in studies that conclude ERT improves depression is the inclusion of women who are suffering significant physical problems associated with menopause.

Women who are sleep-deprived because of frequent hot flashes may feel much less depressed when menopause symptoms ebb naturally[40] or when ERT relieves hot flashes and they are able to sleep through the night.[41] This doesn't prove that ERT treats depression in the absence of other complaints—but it certainly may explain the experience some ERT users have of feeling more energetic.[42]

A report from the randomized PEPI trial found that HRT had little effect on anxiety or affect, even though it did alleviate hot flashes.[43]

Slaven and Lee noted that pre- and postmenopausal women significantly improved their moods with exercise, regardless of HRT status.[44]

Research has focused only minimally on the effect of progestins on mood and depression. However, these few studies suggest that progestins, as a component of combined HRT, may in fact increase depression.[45] Moreover, a 1990 study from England reports a disproportionate number of suicides in women taking HRT and suggests that mood swings may actually be a side effect of long-term use.[46]

Alzheimer's Disease: No Help From HRT

Alzheimer's disease, the most common form of dementia, is a condition of substantial decline in the intellectual abilities of memory, learning, and reasoning.

The disease is a distinct type of dementia difficult to diagnose, and its incidence and prevalence are hard to establish. More women than men are its victims, but that probably is due to women's longer life expectancy and the fact that women survive longer with the disease than do men, on average.[47, 48]

Incidence of diagnosed Alzheimer's disease increases with age, decreases with level of education,[49] and seems to be significantly higher among African Americans and Latinos than among whites in the U.S. population.[50] Political influence by health care providers concerned with their medical careers and by executives looking at the bottom line of drug companies has expanded Alzheimer's identification,[51] so that current medical policy is to make its diagnosis "inclusive" or to apply the diagnosis broadly.[52]

> Incidence of diagnosed Alzheimer's disease increases with age, decreases with level of education, and seems to be significantly higher among African Americans and Latinos than among whites.

Two detailed and comprehensive methodological reviews of the literature on estrogen's effects upon cognition, memory, and dementia (one looking at nineteen studies[53] and the other at twenty-three[54]) have been published. Both conclude that current evidence does not support recommending estrogen for improving cognitive function, nor for preventing, delaying the onset, or improving the effects of dementia, including Alzheimer's disease, in peri- or postmenopausal women.

Virtually everyone agrees that large, long-term, randomized, controlled trials are necessary to resolve the role estrogen may play in preventing loss of cognitive function. The Women's Health Initiative has a mental acuity study underway of three thousand older women to assess effects on mental performance. It will follow these women for six years.[55]

In the meantime, some researchers have conducted smaller, shorter randomized trials with women who are already experiencing Alzheimer's disease in hopes that a benefit will arise more quickly in this population. Three recent trials have all found that ERT does not improve cognitive functioning in women or slow the progression of the disease.[56, 57, 58] Unfortunately, these studies aren't always mentioned by those promoting ERT/HRT for Alzheimer's.

CHAPTER THIRTEEN

Will Hormone Therapy Keep You Young?

It is possible to keep skin, bladder, and sex drive in good shape as you age. The evidence that HRT helps is limited.

Many women hear from their health care providers that ERT will keep them young by preventing wrinkles, toning their bladders, and boosting their sex drives. The evidence for this is mixed.

Several studies have shown that estrogen, usually as an implant or skin patch, increases the collagen content in skin,[1, 2] although other studies have found no such effect.[3]

A large observational study of 3,875 post-menopausal women did find less wrinkling and dry skin in white women who used ERT.[4] African American women in this survey had fewer skin conditions than white women and did not benefit from ERT. No effect was seen on skin aging. The study depended on self-reported estrogen use, and the average age of the women at menopause was around forty-five years, substantially younger than the average.

Henry et al., while finding some benefit of HRT for facial skin, noted no effects upon the number and depth of wrinkles.[5] Castelo-Branco and colleagues did note reduced wrinkles for HRT-using nonsmokers, but no benefit for smokers.[6]

The only reported study of ERT and wound healing compared samples of ten postmenopausal estrogen users, nonusers, and younger women and showed beneficial effects of hormone application to the skin, with potential implication for healing skin ulcers in elderly women.[7]

On the other hand, HRT may be a potential cause of skin-related complications.[8, 9]

None of these studies were double-blind, placebo-controlled, and randomized. Because of these shortcomings in research design, it is impossible to know whether estrogen therapy has a real effect on skin and wrinkles. The best way we know to protect skin is to avoid smoking and excessive exposure to the sun.

> The best way we know to protect skin is to avoid smoking and excessive exposure to the sun.

Urinary Incontinence: Estrogen Doesn't Work

Although estrogen has been used for years in managing urinary incontinence (UI) in women, it is a controversial and understudied treatment. UI is the inability to control urination and usually is a result of problems with the muscles that release urine from the bladder or the nerves that control those muscles. It is much more prevalent in women than men (about 85 percent of those with UI are women) and affects some 11 to 17 million adults in the United States. Prevalence increases with age.

> Women have identified Kegel exercises, bladder retraining, and caffeine restriction as more effective in reducing the severity of UI than biofeedback, ERT, or other drug therapies.

Meta-analyses of controlled clinical trials do not support using estrogen as treatment for UI, although some users may perceive it as beneficial.[10, 11] A relatively large, placebo-controlled, randomized trial followed women for six months and concluded, "It seems unlikely that estrogen has a significant role to play" in postmenopausal stress incontinence.[12] In a small trial, Fantl et al. found that those taking the placebo pill showed the same degree of psychological boost as those taking estrogen.[13] Fewer than ten of the many published studies on this topic are controlled clinical trials.

Other nonsurgical treatments can be effective, however. One small study followed eighty-one elderly Wisconsin women a year after they had undergone nonsurgical treatment for incontinence at a community clinic. The women identified Kegel exercises, bladder retraining, and caffeine restriction as more effective in reducing the severity of UI than biofeedback, ERT, or other drug therapies.[14]

Numerous other studies have found biofeedback to be effective for various forms of UI. (See chapter 16, "Alternatives to Hormone Replacement Therapy.")

Evidence from the HERS trial found that combined hormone therapy actually worsened urinary incontinence in older postmenopausal women.[15] There is some weak evidence that ERT is associated with increased risk for UI.[16] Interestingly, Thom and his associates found that oxytocin, a drug used to increase contractions during labor, is dose-related to the development of UI; multiple exposures to the drug increased the risk later in life.[17]

Given the complexity of this condition and the fact that different women respond to different approaches, we encourage women to consider treatments other than hormones, especially biofeedback, Kegel exercises, bladder retraining, urethral inserts, or nonhormonal drugs.

Better Sex

Women approaching menopause are often faced with warnings that if they don't do something to prevent it, their sex lives will go rapidly downhill. Women hear stories written by other women of vaginas so dry that they feel like sandpaper, orgasms hopelessly out of reach, and even a complete lack of interest in sex.[18] In virtually every story, hormones save the day. Sometimes estrogen pills or cream are what help women have better sex, and, more recently in both the popular press and the scientific literature, testosterone is the hormone that does the trick.[19, 20, 21]

It's hard to deny the reality of women's accounts of their experience with menopause, but what are we to make of stories like these? Do all women have to face a sexless, painful, unsatisfied life after menopause unless they use hormone therapy?

Our answer is no, with the advisory that satisfactory sex after menopause may require some adjustments. First, social issues are tremendously important. American culture values youth. While older men are sometimes perceived as sexy because of their power or prestige, older women are not viewed in the same way. Maintaining a positive self-image as a sexual being is an important goal for older women to strive for despite all the negative messages they receive from society.

The physical changes that come with aging are also important. Both men and women experience declines in levels of hormones associated with sexuality, but women are more likely to experience a rapid drop. A Swedish study that followed 152 women for twelve years found that estrogen levels dropped most quickly in the six months after menopause.[22] Although declining levels of estrogen are not associated with diminished interest in sex, some women do experience vaginal dryness.[23, 24] Vaginal dryness can result in painful vaginal sex, but it can be treated successfully.

As mentioned earlier, women and researchers both report that sexual activity, either alone or with a partner, can maintain vaginal lubrication and elasticity.[25] Many women have found that water-based vaginal lubricants are the only help they need to make sex comfortable. Increasing phytoestrogens in the diet may help (see chapter 7).

Women who are still uncomfortable may turn to estrogen, often in cream form. Estrogen cream works in about two weeks. Once vaginal comfort is restored, women can decrease how often and how much they use and find the minimum dose that meets their needs. Most women find that once or twice a week is usually sufficient.

The Effects of Hormones When Ovaries Have Been Removed

Women who lose ovarian function abruptly, either through treatment for cancer or surgical removal, sometimes have severe symptoms. Many women and even some health care providers don't know that ovaries continue to produce estrogen after menopause and that they are an important source of testosterone. Removing the ovaries, even twenty to thirty years after menopause, cuts testosterone levels in half.[26] This does not mean, however, that women whose ovaries have been removed have no testosterone or estrogen. Many women continue to enjoy sex after losing their ovaries.

Interestingly, it appears that taking ERT pills lowers testosterone levels.[27] So some women who've had their ovaries removed and who are taking ERT may find themselves with extremely low levels of testosterone. Small trials in women who have had their ovaries removed have shown that estrogen plus testosterone leads to improved sex compared with ERT alone, but these trials usually include women who also have sleep deprivation and other vasomotor symptoms of menopause that can interfere with sexual interest and activities.[28]

Research at the Human Sexuality Program in New York found that women who reported a complete loss of interest in sex after losing their ovaries and who also had very low testosterone levels were helped by testosterone supplements.[29] While testosterone replacement in women after removal of the ovaries may be reasonable, testosterone supplements are being promoted for much wider use. We share the concerns of Sadja Greenwood, M.D. and others that long-term use of testosterone therapy may be risky. Until these potential risks are understood, routine or widespread use of testosterone may be unwise.[30]

In men, higher levels of testosterone are associated with a higher risk of cardiovascular disease, but we don't know whether this is true for women.[31] High testosterone levels in men are also associated with prostate cancer and baldness, and again, the implications for women are unknown. We do know that testosterone reduces beneficial HDL cholesterol levels and that when given as a pill, it can have harmful effects on the liver in rare cases. (Testosterone can also be given through injection or pellet, but the dosage is more difficult to control.) Finally, higher than normal levels of testosterone have been associated with breast cancer, although the reason for this is unknown.

> Long-term use of testosterone therapy may be risky. Until potential risks are understood, routine or widespread use of testosterone may be unwise.

PART FOUR

The Truth About Hormones

CHAPTER FOURTEEN

The Studies

Doctors are always changing their minds. First they say one thing, and then they say another. Who knows what's right?

Every time the results of a new study are announced, there's always one cynic in the back of the doctor's waiting room who will tell you that all the study means is that health care providers have changed their minds yet again.

People sometimes feel medicine is so complex and health care providers so whimsical that there's no point trying to figure out what we should do—about anything.

"Whatever we figure out is right today will be wrong tomorrow," people say as they philosophically shrug their shoulders, stick their heads in the sand, and absolve themselves from the responsibility of making their own decisions.

In fact, neither medicine nor health care providers are as contrary as portrayed. The difficulty is that medical research is a process and scientists are constantly making new discoveries. An epidemiologist uncovers an association between one thing and another, and then a researcher launches a pilot study to see if there's anything to it. If there is, another researcher might launch a larger study that examines things a bit longer and in more depth to see if the association still holds up. If it does—and if money can be found—another researcher might launch a fourth study to look at what happens to the association when something is done to a group and then compares it with a similar group to which nothing is done. Finally, another researcher might launch a study that tries to replicate the one just completed. It is at this juncture that most scientists begin to accept that they have found out something new.

Unfortunately, each of these early studies gets reported in the press, often by general assignment reporters who don't know have the training or knowledge to help them evaluate research. They don't know to investigate who funded the study or how to tell if vested interests like drug companies were able to put some spin on the results. What's more, general assignment reporters usually don't know—and aren't given the time by their profit-minded publishers—to check out similar studies so they have a context in which to interpret the findings. The result is that the public hears a different "truth" each time a new study emerges.

> Early studies get reported in the press, often by general assignment reporters who don't have the training to help them evaluate research.

This situation is also what makes books like this necessary to help women make informed choices. We've looked at the major studies on menopause and summarized their findings. We've also presented some context so that you don't walk away from this book thinking we've given you all the answers. Rather, we want you to think of this book as one step in an ongoing process of discovery, testing, and revelation. We urge you to read appendix A, "How to Tell One Study from Another," and then review the following studies carefully. They contain much of what we know of the truth about hormone replacement therapy—as of this moment.

The Nurses Health Study

We refer to the Nurses Health Study often in our book. You have also probably read about it in newspapers and other popular media. Funded primarily by the federal government, it began as an attempt to determine if oral contraceptives increased the risk of breast cancer.

In 1976, 121,700 married nurses, aged thirty to fifty-five, agreed to fill out health questionnaires every two years. This is an observational, prospective, and self-reporting study, and it is much less expensive to do than studies where the researchers talk to every participant. The researchers chose to study nurses because it was believed they would be more motivated to stick with the study for many years and would be familiar with medical terms and able to describe specific health conditions that occurred as they aged.

The Nurses Health Study has now been going on for over twenty years. Recent reports include information on

70,533 postmenopausal participants. With this large number of older women, researchers are able to look for correlations among diet, exercise, hormone use, dietary supplements, and various serious health conditions. The Nurses Health Study provides information on nearly every topic addressed in this book. The two most significant findings are that breast cancer incidence rises with each year of ERT use and that women taking ERT are less likely to die of heart disease.

> The question the Nurses Health Study cannot answer is, Does estrogen make women healthy, or do healthy women take estrogen?

Even though this study is very large and gives us invaluable information on ERT's long-term effects, its findings are not conclusive proof that the choices observed are the actual causes of the health problems of the participants. The question the Nurses Health Study cannot answer is, Does estrogen make women healthy, or do healthy women take estrogen?

Postmenopausal Estrogen/ Progestin Intervention (PEPI)

Unlike the Nurses Health Study, PEPI (pronounced "peppy") is a randomized trial. Nearly nine hundred postmenopausal women volunteered for it. They were screened at the beginning of the study to make sure they had no health problems.

These women were given pills that look exactly alike. They received a placebo, Premarin, Premarin plus Provera every day, Premarin every day plus Provera fourteen days a month, or Premarin plus micronized progesterone. The women took their pills for three years and went regularly for mammograms, endometrial biopsies, cholesterol tests, and bone density measurements.

At the end of three years, the PEPI study found that (1) ERT taken by itself caused endometrial hyperplasia, a risk factor for endometrial cancer; (2) all types of HRT prevented this increased risk; (3) ERT and HRT protect equally against bone loss; (4) ERT and HRT both increased breast density, making mammograms more difficult to read; and (5) ERT alone had a positive effect on cholesterol levels. PEPI also found that the synthetic progestin Provera interfered with this beneficial effect on cholesterol and micronized progesterone did not.

Although this study has a very strong design and its results are reliable, it doesn't provide final answers for women making decisions about ERT/HRT. Its three-year intervention wasn't long enough to determine the effect of hormones on diseases such as breast cancer or heart disease that take many years to develop.

Heart and Estrogen/Progestin Replacement Study (HERS)

Similar to PEPI, the Heart and Estrogen/Progestin Replacement Study randomized women and followed them for four years. The difference is that the researchers recruited 2,763 women who already had heart disease, either a previous heart attack or angina (chest or shoulder pain indicating that the heart isn't getting enough oxygen).

Because these women already had heart disease, it was possible to determine whether or not hormones helped prevent the disease from worsening in a fairly short timeframe. This is unlike PEPI and the Nurses Study, which enrolled women who were not known to have heart disease and in whom it takes many years to determine the effect of hormones on potential heart disease.

> In the first year of the HERS study, the women on Premarin and Provera were more likely to have another heart attack than the women taking the placebo. This effect reversed itself by the fourth year.

Women took either Premarin plus Provera or a placebo and went for regular examinations. HRT did not prevent heart problems. In the first year of the study, the women on Premarin and Provera were more likely to have another heart attack than the women taking the placebo. This effect reversed itself by the fourth year. When the study ended, the number of women experiencing a second heart attack or death was equal in the two groups.

This study is very important because it is the first randomized trial to determine a heart disease outcome. However, in weighing the implications, it's important to remember that the HERS women already had heart disease and that they took combined hormones. The study can't be used to draw conclusions about estrogen used alone or on the effect of HRT on healthy women.

Estrogen Replacement and Atherosclerosis (ERA)

The Estrogen Replacement and Atherosclerosis study is a randomized trial similar to HERS. It recruited women who already had some evidence of heart disease in the form of narrowed arteries/atherosclerosis.

Three hundred and nine women took part in the study. They took Premarin, Premarin plus Provera, or a placebo. The researchers followed them for three years. To assess the progression of their heart disease, the women underwent X-rays that showed whether their coronary arteries continued to narrow. This study is interesting to those who follow women's health because it confirms the results of both PEPI and HERS. ERT and HRT both improved cholesterol levels, just as PEPI had seen in healthy women. However, just as the HERS study found, women taking hormones showed no improvement in their heart disease.

Again, although this study is important and provides conclusive evidence, it only applies to women who already have at least some evidence of heart disease when they begin taking hormones.

Women's Health Initiative (WHI)

The Women's Health Initiative is currently the only ongoing study that provides information for healthy women on the long-term effects of taking hormones for prevention. It's the largest randomized trial of hormones ever attempted.

Twenty-five thousand women are participating. They have been randomly assigned to take either a placebo or hormones. They take HRT if they still have their uterus and ERT if they have had a hysterectomy. The volunteers will take the hormones for at least nine years.

The Women's Health Initiative will reveal the effect of hormones on (1) heart disease and other cardiovascular conditions such as blood clots and stroke; (2) breast, endometrial, colon, and ovarian cancers; (3) Alzheimer's disease; and (4) fractures.

Although this study began in 1993, it took until 1998 to finish recruiting the great number of women needed. It will be 2005 at the earliest before final results are available.

The Women's Health Initiative is currently the only ongoing study that provides information for healthy women on the long-term effects of taking hormones for prevention.

The added strength of the Women's Health Initiative is that, unlike the studies described previously, it includes women of color in numbers proportional to the American population. Its weaknesses are that it is not testing alternative interventions, and the only estrogen in the test is Premarin.

The WHI has already produced results that surprised many proponents of ERT/HRT. It found that the first two years of hormone use increased the risk of heart attack and stroke in women who had been healthy before starting hormones.

Rancho Bernardo Study

We've included the Rancho Bernardo study, a relatively small study of a group of women all very similar to each other, because it is often referred to by health practitioners and reported in the media.

The Rancho Bernardo Study involves women living in a retirement community in Rancho Bernardo, California. It is similar to the Nurses Health Study in that it recruited women who were willing to be followed for many years. However, it's smaller and usually reports on the health experiences of between only eight hundred and a thousand women.

The Rancho Bernardo study has found almost without exception that women taking either ERT or HRT are healthier. They are less likely to be diagnosed with Alzheimer's disease, less likely to die of a heart attack, and less likely to suffer osteoporotic fractures. This study and others like it are often used as "proof" that healthy women who take hormones get results. The weakness is that it only observes women who have chosen to take ERT/HRT. It's not clear whether the hormones themselves cause the women's good health, or if other factors in their lives, such as a health-conscious lifestyle, are responsible.

CHAPTER FIFTEEN

When Is Hormone Therapy Appropriate?

Only you can decide when hormone replacement therapy is appropriate.

We at the National Women's Health Network believe that hormone therapy is useful for those women who experience extreme menopausal discomfort, women who are at high risk of fractures or who have already had a fracture from severe osteoporosis, and some women whose ovaries were removed at a young age.

We also believe estrogen is not an appropriate treatment to prevent Alzheimer's disease or heart disease. Based on the results of the HERS trial, in particular, we believe there is sufficient evidence to recommend that women with a history of heart disease not take hormones.

Finally, we believe that it is inappropriate for clinicians to encourage hormone use in those women experiencing natural menopause without first assessing their individual risks for osteoporosis, heart disease, breast cancer, and endometrial cancer. Risks and benefits must be assessed at different ages as well. We'd like to see clinicians start to offer women other options.

How to Think About Your Risks and Benefits

When women evaluate the potential risks and benefits of estrogen, or estrogen plus a progestin, they often find themselves evaluating the scientific evidence. The lack of evidence from proper clinical trials makes us reluctant to accept some of the alleged benefits of hormone replacement therapy and at the same time makes us question whether some of the alleged risks have been conclusively proven. At this stage in the research, women will have to decide for themselves what to do. Some women are more anxious to avoid possible but not yet proven risks than they are willing to seek out possible but not yet proven benefits.

Some women have permanent conditions that make hormone therapy very important, including surgical removal of the ovaries or long-term use of steroids for treatment of medical conditions. Other women have breast cancer, liver disease, or blood clots that make hormone use especially risky.

Most women will find themselves somewhere in between these clear-cut situations. For these women, evaluating the risks and benefits they perceive for themselves is the most important part of deciding whether to take hormones.

Many risk factors are not absolute. We encourage women evaluating whether hormone therapy is appropriate for fracture prevention to look at the list of risk factors on page 147. We recommend using this list as a guide to making changes that will reduce the chance of fractures and help avoid the unknown risks of hormone therapy.

Women must also consider which of the possible benefits of estrogen are important to them. Health care providers and health policy makers often imply that women are cancer-phobic when they refuse to trade an increased risk of breast cancer for the supposed decrease in heart disease. It is constantly stressed to women that they are much more likely to die of heart disease than cancer. In this area, many women have a commonsense understanding of a little known statistic. The average woman who dies of heart disease loses eight years of life,[1] whereas women who die of breast cancer lose, on average, nineteen years.[2]

> The average woman who dies of heart disease loses eight years of life, whereas women who die of breast cancer lose, on average, nineteen years.

In other words, the risks of ERT/HRT tend to come earlier in life and the benefits—if any—late in life.

What to Take: Estrogen Alone or Combined Hormones?

Women who have had a hysterectomy and face no danger of endometrial cancer are usually advised to take estrogen alone. They should not take combined hormones that, in their situation, offer no known benefits over estrogen alone.

Most clinicians advise a woman who has her uterus to take estrogen and a progestin. The evidence that increased risk of endometrial cancer is reduced by adding a progestin is solid, but the risk of breast cancer does not appear reduced and may be increased.[3]

How to Take ERT/HRT

Pills

Pills are the most common way to take ERT. It is the form taken by women in heart disease studies and nearly all osteoporosis studies.

The most common estrogen pill, Premarin, is a naturally occurring mix of hormones called CEE (conjugated equine estrogens), usually given in a 0.625 mg daily dose. Women who don't get relief from hot flashes at that dose sometimes take higher doses. However, risks increase right along with the dose. Several half-strength doses of estrogen are approved for osteoporosis prevention when taken with extra calcium. Estradiol pills, the most commonly used estrogen in Europe, are available in equivalent doses. Other types of estrogen are less commonly used.

> There are no studies to show whether there are differences in safety among CEE, estradiol, and estrone.

CEE is about half equilin, a horse estrogen, and half estrone, an estrogen common to women and horses. Estradiol is another estrogen manufactured by the human ovary and is also available as pills. Estrone and estradiol convert to one another in the body; a woman who takes one will also increase blood levels of the other. There are no studies to show whether there are differences in safety among CEE, estradiol, and estrone. Estradiol, estrone, and conjugated estrogens are all available as generic medications, but CEE, which contains horse estrogen, is only available in the brand-name Premarin.

The Patch

Available in the United States for the past ten years, the patch is a convenience for many women. It is effective for hot flashes and other complaints and was recently approved for osteoporosis prevention. Estrogen delivered from the patch through the skin does not have the beneficial effect of increasing HDL cholesterol levels. On the other hand, the patch may avoid some complications associated with estrogen pills, such as gall bladder disease, high blood pressure, and blood clots, since it does not have to first pass through the liver (but this has not been proven). The estrogen in the patch is estradiol. Some women complain of skin irritation as a side effect.

Vaginal Cream

Usually used by women whose major menopausal complaint is vaginal dryness, cream is applied directly to the vagina in amounts controlled by the user. Although estrogen in vaginal cream is easily absorbed and distributed throughout the whole body, women can use small amounts every few days and expose themselves to less estrogen than in pills or patches. Some breast cancer survivors who can't find any other way to treat vaginal dryness and must avoid high doses of ERT use this approach. Vaginal estrogen cream can be either CEE or estradiol. There is also an estradiol tablet made for vaginal use and an estradiol-releasing ring that is worn in the vagina.

Pellets

Biodegradable estrogen pellets have been manufactured for many years, but they have never been approved by the FDA. They are inserted in the arm, last for several months, and are a convenient way to get estrogen. However, dosages may vary and send hormone levels far above the normal for premenopausal women.

Progestins

Medroxyprogesterone (Provera and others) is the most commonly used progestin. Doses of 5 to 10 mg taken for at least twelve days in each cycle protect against the risk of endometrial cancer. This schedule usually results in bleeding every month. Some clinicians advocate taking a 2.5 mg dose every day of the month to avoid this withdrawal bleeding. Although progestins protect the uterus, they also seem to partially counteract the HDL cholesterol benefit of estrogen pills.[4]

Combination Products

Several combination products, containing both an estrogen and a progestin, are available in pill or patch form. Combination pills may contain estradiol and ethinyl estradiol as the estrogen and medroxyprogresterone, levonorgestrel, or norethindrone acetate as the progestin. There are no demonstrated advantages in safety or efficacy of one combination product over another, or of combination products over taking estrogen and progestin separately.

CHAPTER SIXTEEN

Alternatives to Hormone Replacement Therapy

You can relieve every single symptom—and prevent heart disease and osteoporosis—without the risks of HRT.

Freddie Ann Hoffman, a physician formerly at the FDA, listens while on her treadmill to a talk show she finds offensive. She finds fury useful fuel to make herself work out harder!

If You Don't Want to Take Hormones

Many women prefer alternative approaches to treating or preventing menopausal symptoms, osteoporosis, and heart disease. If you don't want to take hormones, you may want to carefully review your overall health and risk factors with a supportive health care provider and then consider the alternatives you see here and in the preceding chapters.

Freeze Hot Flashes

Hot flashes are arguably the single symptom that aggravates us the most as we approach menopause. They wake us up from sleep at night and give rise to the stereotype of women becoming "moody" or "grouchy." They distract us both at work and play.

Some lucky women never have hot flashes. Others have them in mild form and infrequently. The worst sufferers live with hot flashes a dozen times a day and feel as though they're living in a sauna.

Many women find ways to handle hot flashes that don't involve HRT. Please remember that what works for one woman may not help another. Here are some of the more popular strategies, along with some studies to help you evaluate their effectiveness.

Breathe   One study compared paced respiration (slow, deep breathing) against muscle relaxation and alpha EEG biofeedback in thirty-three postmenopausal women.[1] Practicing paced respiration for four months reduced the frequency of hot flashes by 39 percent. There was no significant relief from progressive muscle relaxation or biofeedback.

In a more recent trial by the same investigators, twenty-four postmenopausal women with at least five hot flashes a day were randomized to either paced respiration (thirteen women) or biofeedback (eleven women). Paced respiration decreased hot flashes by 44 percent. There was no change in the biofeedback control group.[2]

Move   A Swedish survey of regular exercisers found that moderate to severe hot flashes and sweating were half as common in exercisers than women in the general population.[3] However, this was not a prospective study, and there may be other differences between gym members and other women.

Learn Relaxation Techniques   "Relaxation response" (RR) is a term that describes physiological changes, including slower heart rate and breathing, that are the opposite of the "fight or flight" response.[4] Relaxation response can be invoked by different techniques, like being in a comfortable posture in a quiet room while listening to music or fixing one's gaze to avoid conscious thought. In a randomized, controlled, seven-week study, forty-five women over age forty-four experiencing at least five hot flashes daily were randomized to a relaxation response group, a reading group, or a group that simply kept a record of symptoms experienced.[5] The relaxation group received instruction in RR and practiced the technique twenty minutes daily. The reading group read leisure material for twenty minutes a day. Thirty-three women completed the trial.

Hot flash frequency did not change in any group. Intensity decreased significantly

> Many women make dietary changes and use natural products to relieve hot flashes. Caffeine, chocolate, spicy or hot foods, and alcohol often aggravate hot flashes.

only in the relaxation response group (p<0.05). State anxiety, resulting from a specific situation or stimulus, did not change in any group. Trait anxiety, stemming from personality characteristics, assessed by the Spielberger State-Trait Anxiety Inventory, decreased significantly only in the RR group (p<0.04).

Ditch Foods That Cause Flashes   Many women make dietary changes and use natural products to relieve hot flashes. Caffeine, chocolate, spicy or hot foods, and alcohol often aggravate hot flashes.

Add Foods That Balance Hormones   Others make more major changes in their diets and eat plant foods high in natural weak estrogens, called phytoestrogens. High amounts of phytoestrogens are present in soy products and other legumes (see chapter 7).

Join a Support Group!

Much of the anxiety, depression, irritability, and "moodiness" that we blame on menopause really has little to do with hormones. More often, they are related to women's natural progression through midlife. This is the time when most of us evaluate who we are and what we've done so far with our lives. This is when we figure out who we want to be and what we want to do in the second half of life. Many women find that discussing their menopause issues is a way to break down the isolation they experience and helps them to gain strength.

Stay Cool   Wear and sleep in layers. Shedding clothes quickly can help when your internal temperature rises. Sleeping nude helps to dissipate the heat of night sweats, and several layers of light bedclothes can make it easier to cool off. A portable, battery-powered fan in your office can be a godsend.

Nonhormonal Drugs

There are also pharmaceutical alternatives to estrogen, including renlaxafine (a selective serotonin reuptake inhibitor) and clonidine, which can relieve hot flashes.

Eliminate Vaginal Dryness

Estrogen clearly helps vaginal dryness, but other therapies may work just as well. Here are a few.

Reach for Lubricants   People tend to have strong individual preferences regarding lubricants, so it's best to buy small test sizes to find the best one for you. Some lubricants contain carbopols (Replens is a common brand) that stick to the vaginal cells for days, an effect that can be very useful. It is possible that regular insertion of carbopol-containing vaginal lubricants may be even more helpful in maintaining vaginal health than just using these products before sex.

> People tend to have strong individual preferences regarding lubricants, so it's best to buy small test sizes to find the best one for you.

Some women apply an applicator of carbopols two or three times a week and then use more before sex.

Soothe With Natural Oils   Vaginal dryness and itching can be relieved by applying vitamin E, almond oil, sesame oil, or coconut oil directly to the vagina.

Have Sex   For some women, sex itself improves vaginal comfort. Women who took part in a survey conducted by the Menopause Self Help group in Boston reported that regular sexual activity, either alone or with a partner, helped relieve vaginal dryness and could prevent discomfort during intercourse.[6]

Incontinence Can Be Avoided and Treated

Incontinence is common among women. There are two kinds. The more common is stress incontinence, the loss of urine during coughing, sneezing, or physical exertion. Urge incontinence is involuntary urine loss after a sudden strong urge to urinate. It is common for women to experience a combination of symptoms. Here's what may help.

Kegel   These exercises are so popular that the word "kegel" has become a verb—as in "Have you kegeled today?" No wonder! Kegels are sometimes an effective means of improving control over urination, and they can increase sexual pleasure as well. Kegels are helpful with both types of incontinence.

Chalker and Whitmore, authors of a book on bladder problems, describe how to do these exercises and suggest that users may need to persevere for several months to get results. Here's the exercise: Lying on a floor or bed, successively tighten the vaginal muscles as if you were stopping urine flow, then tighten the muscles of the anus as if you were stopping a bowel movement.[7]

If you are unsure whether you are using the proper muscles, sit on a toilet and try actually stopping and starting urination as you begin to urinate. If you cannot stop urine flow, it means either that your muscles are weak or you are using the wrong ones. To identify the correct muscles, put a finger or two inside your vagina and squeeze the finger(s) with the vaginal muscles. Biofeedback methods may be helpful for those who have difficulty identifying or controlling these muscles on their own.

Once you have identified these two muscle groups, tighten them in turn, pulling upward and inward. Hold these muscles tight, counting slowly to three, breathing slowly and deeply, and then relax. Do this five to ten times several times a day, increasing the number and length of contractions and the number of sets over time. Eventually, you should be contracting the muscles for ten seconds or longer. Alternate sets of these long slow contractions with sets of fast flicks.[8]

Not everyone learns kegeling easily. For some, biofeedback or vaginal weights may be more helpful.

Consider Biofeedback   Biofeedback is a technique that provides you with immediate and observable information about your body's performance. It may be particularly helpful in controlling urge incontinence. A recent well-designed, double-blind, controlled trial found biofeed-back superior to conventional drug treatment for urge incontinence.[9] One hundred ninety-seven women aged fifty-five to ninety-two were randomized to one of three groups: biofeedback, the drug oxybutynin, or placebo.

The biofeedback/behavioral training group went through four training sessions that included identifying and contracting pelvic muscles and "urge strategies." These were sitting down, relaxing, contracting pelvic muscles repeatedly, and proceeding to the toilet at a normal pace once urgency subsided.

Patients kept "bladder diaries." Mainly, they recorded fewer incontinence episodes and perceptions of improvement and satisfaction with the treatments. Biofeedback and behavioral training was significantly

---

Read On!

Several books provide useful information about alternatives to hormone use. We recommend *The New Ourselves, Growing Older*,[10] *Dr. Susan Love's Hormone Book*,[11] *Menopause, Naturally*,[12] *Menopause, Me and You*,[13] *Understanding Menopause, Women and the Crisis in Sex Hormones*, and *Without Estrogen*.[14]

The National Women's Health Network also has a packet of information on alternative remedies for menopausal discomforts. Order at www.womenshealth network.org or through the Women's Health Information Clearinghouse, 514 Tenth Street NW, Fourth Floor, Washington, DC 20004.

more effective and more satisfactory to the patients than drug treatment or taking a placebo. Biofeedback resulted in an 80.7 percent reduction of incontinence episodes, compared to a 68.5 percent reduction with drug treatment and a 39.4 percent reduction with the placebo. In the biofeedback group, 96.5 percent of the patients were comfortable enough with their treatment to continue indefinitely, while only 14 percent wanted to receive another treatment. Although drug treatment was effective, only 54.7 percent of these people stated they could continue it indefinitely, while 75.5 percent stated that they wanted to receive another treatment.

Pelvic floor muscle (PFM) training, the technical term for kegeling, and biofeedback are effective even on homebound elders. One hundred and five homebound adults over sixty were randomized to biofeedback-assisted pelvic floor muscle training or to an untreated control group. The PFM group achieved a 75 percent reduction in urinary accidents, compared to a 6.4 percent reduction in the control group.[15] Those in the control group then received the PFM training. A total of 85 patients completed treatment, achieving a median 73.9 percent reduction in urinary accidents.

For stress incontinence, pelvic floor muscle exercises are effective. However, adding biofeedback to them may not result in any additional improvement. A systematic review of eleven randomized controlled trials found strong evidence for the efficacy of PFM exercises in reducing stress urinary incontinence.[16] However, this review found no evidence that PFM exercises with biofeedback are more effective than PFM exercises alone.

Other "aids" to effective PFM exercising include electrical stimulation and vaginal cones, both of which have been used successfully to treat incontinence. Electrical stimulation requires special equipment and is usually used daily for a thirty-minute session of intermittent vaginal electrical stimulation (individually adapted based on a woman's ability to hold a voluntary contraction.)

Vaginal "cones" are weighted plastic tampon-like devices that are a crude form of biofeedback. Vaginal cones fall out if one is not contracting pelvic muscles adequately. The weights are graduated at 20, 40, and 70 grams, with trainees moving on to heavier ones after successfully retaining the lighter ones. Vaginal cones are now sold directly from catalogs to women.

For stress incontinence, however, all these doodads may be unnecessary. In a single-blind, randomized controlled trial, 107 women with stress incontinence were randomized to pelvic floor exercises, electrical stimulation, vaginal cones, or a control group that was offered a continence guard, a disposable vaginal device that compresses the urethra.[17] Women did the pelvic floor exercises at home (eight to twelve high-intensity contractions three times daily) and in a group setting once weekly with a physical therapist who led them in different positions and included breathing and relaxation exercises.

Researchers calculated pelvic floor muscle strength and did a pad test of standardized bladder volume. This involved emptying the women's bladders by catheter, then refilling them with saline, after which the women wore a preweighed pad and ran in place and performed jumping jacks. The pad was then reweighed. Muscle strength was evaluated by vaginal balloon catheter attached to a transducer. Improvement in muscle strength and reduction in leakage was significantly better after pelvic floor exercises than electrical stimulation or vaginal cones.

The Best Way to Prevent Fractures

The best way to prevent fractures is to prevent falls. Falls are the immediate precipitating factor for approximately 90 percent of hip fractures and 80 percent of other fractures in women.[18]

Minimize Alcohol and Tranquilizers   Use and overuse of alcohol and tranquilizers such as Valium, Dalmane, and Librium and many other medications, including some blood pressure medications and antidepressants, can cause dizziness, lightheadedness, and increased risk of falling.[19, 20, 21] Sidney Wolfe's *Worst Pills, Best Pills* lists fifty-three drugs that can cause falls (see table 16.1).[22]

> Practical ideas like the correct glasses, nonslip rugs, and ice-free sidewalks may prevent more fractures than pharmaceutical interventions.

Prevent Slips   A recent British study compared people who fell and were treated medically with people who fell and were treated by an interdisciplinary approach, including a medical assessment and drug modification as well as fall risk assessment and prevention.[23] The interdisciplinary approach

TABLE 16.1   Drugs That Can Cause Falls*

Brand Name	Generic Name
Heart and blood vessel drugs	
Ismo, Imdur	isosorbide-5-mononitrate
Isordil, Sorbitrate	isosorbide dinitrate
Nitro-Bid, Nitrostat, Transderm-Nitro	nitroglycerin
Mind-affecting drugs	
ANTIDEPRESSANTS	
Asendin	amoxapine
Aventyl, Pamelor	nortriptyline
Desyrel	trazodone
Elavil	amitriptyline
Limbitrol	amitriptyline/chlordiazepoxide
Ludiomil	maprotiline
Luvox	fluvoxamine
Norpramin	desipramine
Paxil	paroxetine
Prozac	fluoxetine
Sinequan	doxepin
Tofranil	imipramine
Triavil	amitriptyline/perphenazine
Wellbutrin	bupropion
Zoloft	sertraline
ANTIPSYCHOTICS	
Compazine	prochlorperazine
Haldol	haloperidol
Mellaril	thioridazine
Navane	thiothixene
Prolixin	fluphenazine
Risperdal	risperidone
Stelazine	trifluoperazine
Thorazine	chlorpromazine
Triavil	amitriptyline/perphenazine
Zyprexa	olanzapine

Brand Name	Generic Name
BARBITURATES	
Burtisol	butabarbital
Luminel, Solfoton	phenobarbital
Nembutal	pentobarbital
TRANQUILIZERS OR SLEEPING PILLS	
Atarax, Vistaril	hydroxyzine
Ativan	lorazepam
BuSpar	buspirone
Centrax	prazepam
Dalmene	flurazepam
Doriden	glutethimide
Halcion	triazolam
Librium	chlordiazepoxide
Miltown, Equanil	meprobamate
Noctec	chloral hydrate
Noludar	methyprylon
Placidyl	ethclorvynol
Restoril	temazepam
Serax	oxezepam
Tranxene	clorazepate
Valium	diazepam
Xanax	alprazolam

Neurological drugs

Dilantin	phenytoin
Klonopin	clonazepam
Luminel, Solfoton	phenobarbital
Tegretol	carbamazepine

Other drugs

Zyban	bupropion

---

* From *Worst Pills, Best Pills 1999*, by Sidney Wolfe (Public Citizen Health Research Group, 1600 20th Street, NW, Washington, DC 20009, cited in Public Citizen Health Research Group's Health Letter 15(4): 1999). Reprinted with permission.

significantly reduced the risks of further falls. Practical ideas like having eye tests and getting the correct glasses, nonslip rugs, getting out of bed slowly, and ice-free sidewalks may prevent more fractures than pharmaceutical interventions.

Wear the Right Shoes   Dr. Carol Frey, director of the Foot and Ankle Center at the Los Angeles Orthopedic Hospital, says avoiding falls is often as simple as choosing the right shoes for different situations. Her research has found that 28 percent of falls in older people come from wearing the "wrong" shoes for the surface where they are: 60 percent of the seniors who were wearing sneakers fell because their shoes caught or dragged on the floor, and 40 percent fell because their shoes were too slippery.[24]

Increase Strength, Agility, and Balance   Exercise also plays an important role in reducing falls. One study found that a home-based exercise program focusing on strength and balance reduced falls and injuries in women eighty and older.[25] The Study of the Osteoporotic Fractures Research Group found physical activity was associated with reduced risk of hip fractures and suggested, "Exercise may reduce the likelihood of falling or may enable a protective response in the event of a fall through enhanced balance, reaction time, coordination, mobility, and muscle strength." After controlling for bone mineral density, hip strength, and the number of falls, they emphasized that the link between physical exercise and reductions in hip fracture relates to many factors and "is not completely explained by its effects on bone mass and muscle strength."[26]

Wear Padding   It is important to plan ahead to reduce injuries if falls do occur. Several studies have found that hip protectors, special tight-fitting padded undergarments that decrease the impact of a fall, significantly reduce hip fractures.[27, 28, 29, 30] The most recent of these studies looked at 1,801 frail but ambulatory adults. One group wore hip protectors, and the other group served as the control. The people wearing hip protectors had a 60 percent reduction in hip fractures, even though they didn't wear them all the time! Nine of the thirteen hip fractures that occurred in that group occurred when the subjects were not wearing their protectors.

Some people are reluctant to wear special undergarments, finding them uncomfortable or inconvenient. In November 2000, the *New England Journal of Medicine* editorialized in support of their use, calling them "a breakthrough in fracture prevention" and advocated further research into ways to improve the acceptability of these low-tech devices.[31]

Boost Calcium Intake   Lifelong adequate calcium intake can lead to optimum bone mineral density. Postmenopausal calcium intake from diet or supplements may delay bone loss and reduce fractures. In a study believed to be the first to look at both lifelong and current calcium intake in normal postmenopausal women not taking estrogens, researchers found a protective effect on bone density in women who reported high calcium intake, both throughout their lifetime and currently.[32]

Calcium supplements are important, particularly for women who do not eat as many calcium-containing foods as they should. Calcium supplements can reduce bone loss.[33, 34, 35, 36] Women with an average intake of less than 400 mg of dietary calcium each day were able to significantly reduce their bone loss by taking 500 mg calcium citrate or calcium malate.[37] There are different forms of calcium supplements, some more expensive than others. The cheapest, calcium carbonate, is well absorbed except by those with low levels of stomach acid. There is no advantage to more expensive forms. In addition, many nutritional supplements containing combinations of vitamins and minerals are promoted for bone health. These combination supplements, besides being unproven, are much more expensive than basic calcium carbonate.

As we have said throughout this book, low bone mineral density is not the same as fracture risk. Some studies show that women who eat diets rich in calcium lose less bone and are less likely to fracture. A fourteen-year study of older men and women found that hip fractures occurred less in those whose diets contained moderate amounts of calcium.[38] Studies have also found significantly fewer nonvertebral fractures in older women who take both calcium and vitamin D supplements.[39, 40]

Join a Women's Health Group

Join other women and become a member of a local or national women's health group to examine pronouncements from the medical profession, the government, and the pharmaceutical industry. Help challenge those who provide misinformation.

Other studies question the benefits of dietary calcium or calcium supplements for reducing bone loss or risk of fractures in postmenopausal women. The PEPI study showed that in 875 healthy early postmenopausal women higher dietary calcium intake was significantly associated with higher bone mass density of the lumbar spine and total hip. Conversely, the PEPI study found that taking calcium in a supplement rather than in foods was associated with lower bone density. The researchers hypothesized that

> There are different forms of calcium supplements. The cheapest, calcium carbonate, is well absorbed except by those with low levels of stomach acid. There is no advantage to more expensive forms.

this might be related to the fact that women with lower bone density may be more likely to use calcium supplements than women with higher bone density.[41]

The Nurses Health Study showed that higher consumption of dietary calcium did not reduce fractures among middle-aged women.[42, 43] In fact, this study revealed a higher incidence of hip fractures in the group with the highest milk intake. This apparent contradiction may be explained by the role of "calcium wasters" in the diet (see "Avoid Calcium 'Wasters'" on page 249).

Differently designed studies give somewhat different results. In a pro-hormone environment, the media tends to pay more attention to studies that show the limitations of calcium. Thus, it is particularly useful to look at the overall direction of many calcium studies. The excellent review article, "Calcium for Prevention of

Osteoporotic Fractures in Postmenopausal Women" by Robert G. Cumming and Michael C. Nevitt, summarizes results from fourteen studies of calcium supplements (including four randomized trials), eighteen studies of dietary calcium and hip fracture (no randomized trials), and five studies of dietary calcium and other fracture sites (no randomized trials) published between 1966 and early 1997. Using meta-analysis techniques and combining information from many studies, these authors found that 1000 mg per day of dietary calcium was associated with a 24 percent reduction in hip fracture risk:

> Our conclusion is that calcium supplements and dietary calcium probably reduce the risk of osteoporotic fractures in older women. The consistency in effect size between small, randomized trials and the pooled observational studies (after adjustment for measurement error) is particularly impressive. Our systematic review of the evidence supports the current clinical and public health policy of advising women to increase their calcium intake.[44]

Help Your Body Absorb Calcium   Vitamin D is essential for calcium absorption. Women with low blood levels of vitamin D are at significantly increased risk of hip fracture.[45] Understanding how nutrients interact with each other (in this case, calcium and vitamin D) is essential for determining optimum nutrition, but the complexity of designing studies to look at important interactions necessarily limits what can be claimed for individual dietary components.

In their excellent review of thirty years of major calcium studies, Cumming and Nevitt report that the largest (3,270 women) randomized study of calcium and nonvertebral fracture found after eighteen months that high calcium intake was associated with a 27 percent reduction in risk of any nonvertebral fracture and a 27 percent reduction in hip fractures. However, they also note, "Unfortunately, the interpretation of this trial with respect to the effect of calcium is complicated . . . by cointervention with vitamin D."[46] This is because the subjects given calcium were also given vitamin D daily, and that limits what the researchers can say about calcium. It helps women know that "appropriate" amounts of both calcium and vitamin D are important!

Head for the Produce Aisle   Fresh produce contains magnesium and boron, both of which help your body use calcium. One study found that boron has an effect on the body's ability to retain calcium. Twelve women receiving extra boron excreted less calcium and showed higher levels of circulating estrogen.[47] The best sources of natural boron—and good sources of magnesium as well—are apples, pears, grapes, leafy vegetables, nuts, and legumes.

Avoid Calcium "Wasters"   There is plenty of evidence that Western/industrialized lifestyles and diets contribute to the prevalence of osteoporosis. One anthropologist has described people living traditional lifestyles in other parts of the world as "almost immune" to osteoporosis.[48] Western diets foster the development of osteoporosis by not providing enough calcium in the first place and, just as important, by "wasting" the calcium that is ingested.

T. Colin Campbell, a professor of nutritional biochemistry at Cornell University, argues that Americans don't need more calcium; they need less protein. "Studies that have compared fracture rates in different countries against calcium intake have found that the higher the calcium intake, the higher the fracture rates. . . . When you compare dairy food intake against fracture rates, the higher the dairy food intake, the higher the fracture rates. . . . Protein in general and animal protein specifically, when consumed in high quantities, cause a loss of calcium from the body."[49]

Consumption of meat increases the acid load in our bodies and triggers the release of calcium and phosphates from bone in order to buffer the acid. Some researchers believe that milk protein probably does not cause a loss of calcium, but it sometimes appears so, because diets high in milk are often also high in meat.

Studies do show that the closer people get to a plant-based diet, the lower their rates of osteoporosis.[50] A 1992 review of thirty-four published studies compared fracture rates in sixteen countries and found that the higher the animal protein intake, the higher the rate of fracture.[51] Another study found that vegetarians had higher bone density at age seventy than meat eaters at age fifty.[52] Important though these studies are, it is necessary to keep in mind that their results may be influenced by other habits common to vegetarians and those who live in regions where plant-based diets are more common. Often, people with healthful diets also exercise more, which contributes to bone strength.

The typical Western diet encourages a heavy imbalance in the ratio of phosphorus to calcium, and that can cause a loss of bone calcium. The lower the calcium to phosphorous ratio, the less calcium is available. Liver, chicken, beef, pork, and fish, in that order, have the worst calcium to phosphorous ratios. Fruits and vegetables, though lower in calcium, make it more available to the bones because of their "good" calcium to phosphorous ratios.[53] The ratio in milk and eggs is much better than meat products but not as good as fruits and vegetables.[54]

Carbonated beverages are another villain in the American diet. These drinks are a major contributor to the poor calcium to phosphorous ratio consumption in the United States. Carbonated beverage consumption in the United States is about 40 gallons per person per year. A single canned soft drink yields 26 to 76 mg of phosphorus. Add this to our estimated 1430 to 1520 mg of phosphorus from unprocessed foods and 500 to 1000 mg from processed foods for each of us every day, and the phosphorus total is surprisingly high.[55, 56] However, the Rancho Bernardo Study found that a modest intake of carbonated beverages did not appear to have an adverse effect on bone mineral density.[57]

Calcium wasters may be most important in younger women, when peak bone mass is being built. Noting the public health consequences of their research, Grace Wyshak and Rose E. Frish have found a significant association between the consumption of nonalcoholic carbonated beverages and bone fractures in both white middle-class girls aged eight to sixteen and in older women aged twenty-one to eighty who were former college athletes.[58, 59]

Stay Away From Tobacco Smoke   Cigarette smoke can reduce bone mass and delay the healing of fractures.[60] Aside from its other detrimental effects on lungs and heart, smoking may bring on early menopause and increase the severity of menopausal changes.[61]

Go Easy on Caffeine and Alcohol   High levels of caffeine and alcohol significantly contribute to excessive bone loss.[62, 63]

Forget Salt   Increased sodium intake causes an increase in urinary calcium losses, so the high salt intake in the United States is also contributing to osteoporosis.

Be Physically Active   Exercise slows bone loss.[64, 65, 66, 67, 68, 69] The PEPI study found that even moderate levels of leisure time physical activity are positively associated with a beneficial effect on bone mass. The study compared four levels of leisure activity and found a graded effect of leisure activity on bone mass. The levels are:

- Inactive: spends most waking hours either sitting or standing quietly
- Light: leisurely rides a bicycle, does light industrial work or teaching, or light housework
- Moderate: brisk walking, light building, mail carrying, moderate gardening, or home repairs
- Heavy: jogging, high intensity aerobics, strenuous farm work or gardening

"BMD was about 2 to 3 percent higher for each increasing level of leisure activity. . . . From a public health perspective, the benefit conferred by mild and moderate exercise, although lesser in magnitude than that of strenuous exercise, is equally important," writes G.A. Greendale in the *Journal of Women's Health*.[70]

Weight-bearing exercise stimulates bone formation but is less effective than estrogen. However, recent research has found that calcium supplements, combined with moderate exercise programs, can slow bone loss more effectively than either one alone.[71, 72] A randomized, prospective study of forty white women aged fifty to seventy demonstrated the many health benefits of a strength-training program comprised of two forty-five-minute sessions each week for one year. The program not only improved strength, but it also improved bone mineral density, muscle mass, and balance, and spontaneously increased other weekly physical activity in the exercise group.[73] Any bone gained by exercise, however, will be lost when the exercise program stops. Use it or lose it!

> In addition to other health benefits, such as cardiovascular health, exercise improves strength, bone mass, muscle mass, balance, and flexibility—all factors that relate to the prevention of osteoporosis and fractures.

In emphasizing the significance of exercise, it is important to note that in addition to other health benefits, including cardiovascular health, exercise improves strength, bone mass, muscle mass, balance, and flexibility—all factors that relate to the prevention of both osteoporosis and fractures. In contrast, hormones and other drug interventions only improve bone mass and have no effect on other factors that may reduce fractures.

Prevent Heart Disease

Study after study has shown that heart disease is largely preventable through a concerted program of diet and exercise. Here are some of the strategies that are responsible for reducing heart disease in the United States by a whopping 28 percent since 1963.

Zap Total Fat   Reduce the fat in your diet to 20 percent or less of total calories. The benefits of a moderately low-fat diet (30 percent or less) for heart disease prevention have been proven, and diets containing less than 20 percent may be even more beneficial.

Cut Saturated Fat   Reduce consumption of high-fat animal foods, including whole milk dairy products, soft cheeses, butter, eggs, red meat, and other high-fat meats such as bacon, luncheon meat, and frankfurters.

Substitute "Good" Fat for "Bad" Fat   Use monounsaturated oils (olive, canola, or peanut) in moderation and in place of both polyunsaturated fats and hydrogenated fats—both of which generate artery-clogging transfatty acids. Avoid margarines altogether unless the label says they are free of transfatty acids.

Lessen Stress   Personality and lifestyle factors make a difference. A driven, Type A personality, hostility, depression and anxiety, lack of job control, and lack of social support are all linked to the risk of coronary heart disease.[74] Taking charge of your life and reducing these negatives decrease your risk of heart disease.[75, 76]

Substitute Soy for Meat   Soy intake appears to lower cholesterol levels. An analysis of thirty-eight controlled clinical trials found that eating an average of 47 grams of soy protein (about one and a half ounces) daily was associated with reducing total cholesterol by 9.3 percent, reducing LDL by 12.9 percent, and reducing triglycerides by 10.5 percent. There was no effect on HDL.[77]

Consider Vitamin E   The evidence supporting this alternative is not as strong as the previous suggestions, but there are some indications that vitamin E may be helpful in reducing the risk of heart disease. In the Nurses Health Study, women who consumed the highest amount of dietary vitamin E had a 34 percent reduction of major coronary disease compared with those with the lowest intake. Those who took vitamin E supplements for more than two years also experienced a reduction in coronary disease risk.[78] But remember, this is an observational study.

Consider the B Vitamins   Homocysteine, a derivative of the amino acid methionine found mainly in animal products, accumulates in the blood and has been linked to an increased risk of cardiovascular disease[79, 80, 81] and stroke.[82] Getting rid of it requires vitamin B_{12}, B_6, and folic acid. People deficient in any of these have higher homocysteine concentrations. Folic acid clearly lowers homocysteine in the blood.[83] Although folic acid is found in fresh fruits and vegetables, few people in this country eat enough of this food group. In the Nurses Health Study, 13 to 15 percent of women twenty to forty-four years of age were deficient in folate.[84]

Get Your Body Moving   Exercise is essential for physical, mental, and emotional vitality. Humans are no more designed to sit in traffic or in front of a computer screen than fish are designed just to tread water or birds solely to perch. Not only is regular exercise associated with lower mortality rates, but also consistent exercise decreases rates of diabetes, hypertension, osteoporosis, and myocardial infarction. It can also lessen stress and sleep disorders.[85]

> Most people spend ten to fifteen hours daily sitting in a car, at a desk or computer terminal, and watching television.

Despite concerted public health campaigns, however, most of us are bigger couch potatoes than ever. More than 60 percent of adults do not exercise consistently, and 25 percent spend none of their leisure time in physical activities. Most people spend ten to fifteen hours daily sitting in a car, at a desk or computer terminal, and watching television.[86]

Sedentary women are twice as likely as active women to have a heart attack. The relative risk of inactivity and coronary heart disease ranges from 1.3 to 1.9. Total physical activity is inversely related to the risks of fatal CHD and first myocardial infarction.[87]

Exercise that is fun is the easiest to do consistently. The exercise that is right for you may be something you have not yet tried. Activities like ballroom, folk, and salsa dancing, aerobics, or African dance can become social events as well as being good for us. Hatha yoga, t'ai chi, and qi gong are gentle exercises that are doable by those with physical limitations or who are out of shape.

Women who played sports earlier in their lives but whose work and/or family obligations have interrupted their athletic endeavors might try reconnecting with their former sport.

For those who have always aimed to be as inactive as possible, different strategies may be needed. Starting an exercise program at a feasible level is essential for eventual success, and unrealistic goals need to be discouraged. Set low goals like committing to a few minutes of exercise per day. Or try regular walking, which is easy, inexpensive, and most people can do it.

> Many people do better when they ritualize exercise and include other people, whether family, friends, or strangers.

Figure out "when and where" options for yourself. Consider the high school track near home or work, an after-dinner stroll with a spouse or a neighbor, or become a mall walker. (One woman we know, a sixty-five-year-old Japanese American woman with diabetes and foot problems, just passed her 400-mile mark at a shopping mall.)

Many people do better when they ritualize exercise and include other people, whether family, friends, or strangers. Showing up for Jazzercise or an aerobics class three times a week is often easier than deciding each day when and where to exercise.

Three ten-minute sessions a day provide almost identical improvements in fitness, cardiovascular risk, body weight, and fat stores as a continuous thirty-minute workout.[88]

Even in the extremely frail, exercise can have very positive effects. A study of ten nursing home residents, aged eighty-six to ninety-six, indicated that in eight weeks of weight lifting, strength increased 174 percent, walking speed increased 48 percent, and lower extremity strength increased by 61 to 374 percent![89]

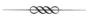

How to Tell One Study From Another

This appendix explains the terminology used when discussing scientific experiments. It may be helpful to readers who are not familiar with the vocabulary of clinical trials and other scientific research. It has been reprinted with permission from Alternative Medicine: What Works, *by Adriane Fugh-Berman, M.D. (Lippincott, Williams and Wilkins, 1997).*

S ome of the terms you'll come across repeatedly in this book may be unfamiliar to you. It's worth learning them, since they're universally used to explain the results of scientific experiments, and knowing them will not only help you read this book but will also stand you in good stead when you read about scientific experiments elsewhere.

Fortunately, scientific terminology isn't hard to learn. That doesn't mean you're going to remember every single term after reading this chapter once. Just let whatever sticks in your mind stick, and ignore the rest. Then, when you encounter a term you're not sure about, refer back to this chapter or look it up in the index. (I've boldfaced the terms where they're defined in this chapter, to make them easy to find.)

Study is a very broad term that covers almost everything that's looked at objectively. A human participant in a study—that is, one of the people whose responses, reactions, or whatever are being studied—is called a **subject.**

A **case study** is a report on one unusual subject by a doctor. Both case studies and stories that patients report themselves are called **anecdotal evidence.** Doctors joke that if we see two cases, we say we're seeing something "time after time," and if we see three cases, we call it a **case series.** Joking aside, a case series should consist of at least five cases. Case series are useful for indicating that something interesting is going on that may merit more formal study.

A **survey** is a kind of study that reports the results of interviewing people on whom no **intervention** is done. (Compare *trial* on page 262.) Since nothing new—no new drug, procedure, dietary restriction, or whatever—is given to them or done to them, we say surveys are **observational.** Surveys simply try to discover how common a disease, treatment, condition, or behavior is—or what **correlations,** or **associations,** there may be between various diseases, behaviors, and so on. (There's a subtle distinction between a *correlation* and an *association* that isn't worth going into here.)

A **positive correlation** means that the more you have of A, the more you have of B. A **negative** (or **inverse**) **correlation** means that the more you have of A, the less you have of B. So, for example, there's a positive correlation between a high-fat diet and heart disease (the more fat you eat, the greater your chance of getting heart disease) and a negative correlation between eating broccoli and getting certain cancers (the more broccoli you eat, the smaller your chance of getting these cancers).

Correlations can't prove anything absolutely. For example, just because an increased number of storks in an area coincides with an increased number of births, that doesn't prove that storks bring babies.

How many people have a given condition at a given point in time is called its **prevalence** (for example, the number of color-blind people per 100,000 in the United States today or the number of people who were carrying tuberculosis bacteria on January 1, 1900). How many new cases of a condition occur over a given period of time is called its **incidence** (for example, the number of babies born in a given year who are color-blind or the number of new TB cases in the last month). The study of prevalence and incidence falls into the field of **epidemiology,** which looks at patterns of disease and the factors that influence those patterns.

A **retrospective study** looks to the past for clues— you start with the disease and try to find out what caused it. For example, retrospective studies found that the prevalence of cigarette smoking among patients with lung cancer was higher than the prevalence of cigarette smoking among people without lung cancer. (Since you can't intervene in the past, all retrospective studies are observational.)

Retrospective studies can be large or small. To improve their quality, the **case-control** method is often used. This means that, when comparing a group with the disease to a group without it, the two groups are matched as closely as possible with regard to factors like age, sex, geographic location, or any other variable that might affect the likelihood of getting the disease. The perfect case-control study would be of a group of identical twins where one twin in each pair developed a disease and the other twin in each pair didn't.

A **prospective study** is one in which subjects are followed forward in time instead of backward. Unlike retrospective studies, prospective studies can be either observational or interventional. Two famous prospective trials are the Nurses Health Study, in which about 100,000 nurses have been answering annual questionnaires since 1976, and the Health Professionals Follow-up Study, in which about

50,000 physicians and other health professionals have been answering annual questionnaires since 1986.

By analyzing their responses, many associations have been discovered, including the positive correlation between hormone replacement therapy and breast cancer (that is, hormone replacement tends to increase one's risk of getting breast cancer) and the negative correlation between vitamin E intake and cardiovascular disease (that is, taking vitamin E tends to decrease heart disease risk).

Unlike a survey, a **trial** is a study in which the subjects receive an experimental intervention. Since you can only intervene in the present, not in the past, trials are always prospective. A **clinical trial** is one in which the subjects are human—as opposed to **preclinical trials** that use animals, bacteria, cells, and so on.

In a **controlled trial,** at least two groups are compared. The **treated** or **experimental** group receives the intervention, while the other—called the **control group,** or simply the **control**—doesn't. Or different groups may receive different interventions. The groups studied in a trial are also called **arms.**

In a **placebo-controlled** trial, an inactive pill or procedure—the **placebo**—is given to the control group. *Placebo* is Latin for "I will please [you];" placebos got that name because any intervention, including simple attention, tends to make people feel better. Certain conditions, such as headaches, arthritis, and hot flashes, are particularly responsive to placebos—as are some individuals.

Overall, the average **placebo effect** is an astonishing 33 percent (although it can range from much lower to much higher). In other words, an average of a third of the subjects in clinical trials will report significant improvement simply from being given a sugar pill (or some other placebo). So to demonstrate that a treatment works, you have to show that it does significantly better than the placebo that's given to the control group.

A **randomized** trial is one in which subjects are assigned to different groups as randomly as possible—by flipping a coin or using a random number generator. If the researcher decides which subjects go into which group, or if the subjects assign themselves, intentional or unintentional **bias** can creep in and the groups may no longer be comparable (all the sicker patients might end up in one group, for example).

A **crossover** trial is one in which each patient is in each group at different times. For example, group A starts on drug X, and group B starts on the placebo; then, midway through the trial, the subjects are crossed over to the other arm (group A starts taking the placebo and group B starts taking the drug).

Blinding (sometimes, but less frequently, called **masking**) means that the researchers and/or the subjects don't know which group each subject is in. In a **single-blind** study, the subjects don't know, but the researchers do (theoretically, it could also mean that the subjects know and the researchers don't, but there wouldn't be much point to that). Most nonsurgical studies are at least single-blind, since subjects' knowing whether they're getting an experimental treatment or a placebo is obviously likely to affect their responses.

In a **double-blind** study, neither the researchers nor the subjects know which group the subjects are in; all information is coded, and the code isn't broken until the end of the trial. (An exception is made when the difference between the two groups is so pronounced—everyone in the control group is dying, say, and everyone in the treated group is getting well—that it would be unethical to continue to deny the treatment to the controls.)

Double-blinding is important because researchers can give subtle, unconscious cues that can change subjects' responses quite independently of the treatment being tested. If the researchers don't know who's getting the treatment and who's getting the placebo, they can't put out those signals.

Saying that a treatment worked in 50 percent of the subjects tested obviously means a lot more if you're talking about two thousand subjects than if you're talking about two. So a good researcher involves statisticians before a trial begins in order to determine the **sample size** (the number of subjects) that will be necessary to show that the results are **statistically significant**—that is, unlikely to be due to chance.

Statistical significance isn't black and white; it's a matter of degree—what are the *odds* that this result was due to chance? It's measured by something called the **p value** (the *p* stands for "probability"). P values look like this: <.1, <.05, <.01, and so on (< means "less than"). To translate a p value into English, move the decimal point two spaces to the right and say "percent."

A p value of <.01 means that the probability that the results occurred by chance is less than 1 percent. That's a good study. A p value of <.1 means that the probability that the results occurred by chance is less than 10 percent. That isn't so great, since it means that there's almost one chance in ten that the results are meaningless. In general, a p value of <.05 is considered statistically significant.

A large sample size helps to control for **confounding variables** (also called **confounding factors,** or simply **confounders**). For example, a small trial on cardiovascular disease might happen to have a larger number of smokers in one group than the other. In this case, smoking would be a confounding variable, since it's known to cause cardiovascular disease.

If the sample size is large enough, however, one can assume that known—and unknown—confounders will be evenly distributed between the groups. To see why this is, imagine flipping a coin. If you flip it ten times, there's a reasonable chance it will come up heads 70 percent of the time (seven heads, three tails). If you flip it a thousand times, there's almost no chance it will come up heads 70 percent of the time (700 heads, 300 tails).

To put all this together—the gold standard for medical research is a prospective, randomized, double-blind, placebo-controlled trial with a sample size large enough to produce a p value of <.05 or lower. It's useful to know what the gold standard is, because everything—including trials of conventional medical therapies—should be held up to it. (Studies that don't meet the standard aren't necessarily wrong, but they're not proof. Future trials should adhere to the gold standard as much as possible.)

There are just a few more terms you should know. A **meta-analysis** is a relatively new kind of study in which you combine the results from a number of selected trials in order to come to some general conclusions. Meta-analyses are usually done when a number of small trials give ambiguous, conflicting, or statistically insignificant results. When all of the decent trials are combined, there may be enough subjects in the combined treatment group to reach a statistically significant conclusion.

Let's say we're doing a survey of weights in a tiny village that has just eleven inhabitants. There are five children, who weigh 40, 50, 65, 65, and 65 pounds (the last three are triplets); three women, who weigh 105, 115, and 125 pounds; and three men, who weigh 150, 160, and 840 pounds (this last guy has a hormonal disorder).

If we add up all the weights, we get 1,780 pounds; if we divide that by 11, we get 162 pounds. This is the **mean**—it's what we're talking about when we use the word "average" in everyday speech. But it would be very misleading to say that the average person in this village weighs 162 pounds, since all but one of the inhabitants weigh less than that. To deal with situations like this, statisticians have come up with two other kinds of averages—the *median* and the *mode*.

The **median** is the value in the middle of the distribution—the one halfway between the bottom and the top. In this particular example, the median—105 pounds—gives a much better idea of the average weight than does the mean.

The **mode** is the value that occurs most frequently; in this example, it would be 65 pounds (the triplets). In some distributions, the mode is a better indication of what's representative than either the mean or the median.

The **FDA** (the Food and Drug Administration, a regulatory agency of the federal government) requires specific kinds of trials on human subjects before it will approve new drugs. (Animal studies and the like have typically been done before these trials take place.) A **Phase I** trial simply tests for safety; it's usually done on healthy volunteers, without a control group.

In a **Phase II** trial, the drug is given to people with the condition or disease to be treated; it supplies some preliminary data on whether the treatment works and supplements the safety data of the Phase I trial. Phase II trials may or may not use a control group.

A **Phase III** trial assesses efficacy, safety, and dosage, compared with standard treatments or a placebo. Phase III trials are usually randomized and controlled.

Phase I, II, and III trials are usually performed as part of an **IND** (an investigational new drug application to the FDA). After the Phase III trial is completed, the manufacturer can submit an **NDA** (a new drug application), which requests permission to market the drug.

Not routinely required, **Phase IV** studies are done after drugs are approved by the FDA and can be sold to the public. They're randomized trials or surveys that attempt to evaluate long-term benefits and risks.

Finally, *in vitro* (literally, "in glass") refers to studies done in artificial environments like test tubes, and *in vivo* refers to studies done in living organisms.

How to Talk to Your
Health Care Provider

You and your health care provider may be coming from two very different places when the issues of drugs and menopause arise. You may have come in for a regular health checkup and assurance that "all is well." In contrast, your age may be a trigger for your health practitioner to follow the perimenopause or menopause protocol provided by drug companies.

As this book has described, most health practitioners are likely to have been significantly influenced by drug-industry-created "knowledge." As a result, their conversation with you may be based on the assumption that most menopausal women should be offered drug treatment. Flow charts, such as the one shown in figure A2.1, show how physicians learn to counsel their perimenopausal and menopausal patients about what form of treatment to take, not whether to take treatment. The article accompanying this flow chart reminds physicians, "The decision to use hormone supplementation is ultimately the patient's," but then immediately offers guidance for the practitioner about factors that influence patient decisions "to understand the reasons behind the initiation, cessation, or refusal of HRT use."

FIGURE A2.1   HRT Counseling Algorithm

STEP 1—Agenda

- Establish the reason for this visit
- Assess the patient's menopausal status
- **CONSIDER:** Is this an appropriate time to initiate or continue a discussion about perimenopause or menopause?
  - Symptoms
  - Age
  - History

If yes, continue . . .

- Assess patient's current emotional status
  - What is going on in her life?
  - How she feels about it
  - How she is handling it

STEP 2—Initiate Discussion

- **INQUIRE:** "How do you picture yourself in 10 or 15 years?"
- **INQUIRE:** "What do you think is happening in your body during menopause?"
  - Natural process/part of aging
  - Time when physical and emotional changes associated with menopause occur
  - End of menstruation
  - Natural loss of ovarian estrogen and progesterone production
- **INQUIRE:** "How do you view menopause?"
  - Benefits
  - No more periods, no need to worry about contraception
  - Marks a new life phase
  - Common symptoms
    - Hot flushes
    - Night sweats/cold sweats

FIGURE A2.1 HRT Counseling Algorithm (continued)

- Headache
- Mood changes
- Painful intercourse, dry vagina, decreased sex drive
- Difficulty in urination/urinary incontinence
- Potentially increased health risks
  - Cardiovascular disease
  - Osteoporosis
  - Cognitive impairment
- **INQUIRE:** "What sources of information have you seen or used about menopause and/or HRT?"

STEP 3—Assess Readiness and Appropriateness

- **INQUIRE:** "What do you know or think about HRT? Have you considered using HRT? Why or why not?"
  - Reasons why HRT may be considered
    - Relief from menopausal symptoms
      - Hot flushes and other vasomotor symptoms, sleep disturbances, headaches, mood changes
      - Urogenital symptoms (vaginal dryness, vaginal atrophy, sexual dysfunction)
    - Osteoporosis and bone fracture prevention
    - Primary prevention of heart disease
    - Decrease in urinary tract infections and improvement in urgency
    - Possible improved cognition and memory
  - Reasons for NOT wanting HRT
    - Patient does not want to "take drugs"
    - Patient feels that not enough is known about long-term use
    - Articles in the news about risks of HRT have caused substantial worry
    - Therapy may not be convenient

(continued)

FIGURE A2.1 HRT Counseling Algorithm (continued)

- – Patient has received negative information from friends and/or family

- – Fear of cancer

- – Menopause is "natural process not requiring intervention"

- ■ **INQUIRE:** "What do you know/believe about the risks of HRT?"

- • Potential side effects

  - – Cyclic or breakthrough bleeding, menstrual-like symptoms

  - – Breast tenderness, bloating

  - – Irritability (usually improved, but may increase)

  - – Clotting disorders are rare but important to discuss in high-risk patients

  - – Small possible increase in breast cancer risk after long-term use (>5 years)

  - – Gallbladder disease

STEP 4—Assist

- ■ In addition to ERT/HRT, what else can the patient do to protect herself?

  - • Stop smoking

  - • Manage weight

  - • Exercise daily

  - • Eat a healthy diet (e.g., cholesterol, alcohol intake)

  - • Take calcium

  - • Prevent or treat osteoporosis

  - • Prevent falls

  - • Get regular mammograms and do breast self-exam

  - • Screen and manage cholesterol

  - • Screen for and manage hypertension

  - • Use seat belts

FIGURE A2.1 HRT Counseling Algorithm (continued)

- Personalize benefits and potential risks of treatment
- Present treatment options and recommendations
  - Types of treatments
  - Dosage forms: oral, transdermal, vaginal, injectable
    - Low-dose oral contraception (for perimenopausal women) provides contraception, cycle regulation, and symptom relief
    - Regimen: cyclic, continuous, pulsed
    - Duration: short term, long term
- **INQUIRE:** "Do you have any other questions?" Such as:
  - "Are natural products better?"
  - "How long should I take it?"
  - "What other benefits are possible from HRT?"
  - "Will I ever be able to stop HRT? Why or why not?"

STEP 5—Follow-up

- **CONSIDER:** What menopausal symptoms might she experience (e.g., hot flashes), and how long will it take to suppress them?
- **CONSIDER:** What should she do if they cause a problem?
  - Discuss timing for the next health care provider contact
  - Establish a procedure for contact to discuss any issues that arise
  - Re-evaluate the decision whether or not to use HRT
  - Encourage her to contact health care provider before discontinuing HRT
  - Discuss self-management strategies for relief of vasomotor symptoms

Supplement, November 2000. Annenberg Center for Health Sciences at Eisenhower. Supported by an educational grant from Wyeth-Ayerst Laboratories.

This certainly reflects the attitude that drugs are the expected "choice" and does nothing to validate that menopause is a normal, healthy transition for most women. In addition to feeling they need information to make wise decisions about treatment, women often feel on the defensive and need the information to justify why they do not want to take hormones.

A Little Help From Your Friends

We hope this book helps you find the information you need to make informed decisions and to feel good about whatever decision you make. To help you work with your practitioner and get the care you deserve, we've developed a list of situations women frequently encounter. Following each situation is our suggested approach.

Your health care provider makes you feel you are silly to be worrying about the breast cancer risk of hormones or tells you that you should be more worried about heart disease than breast cancer.

Women tell us this all the time! Most health practitioners have never pulled together the "big picture" of women's health in the way we have in this book, because much of their information comes from a manufacturer pushing a particular product for a particular disease. In the last decade, when drug companies consistently pushed the message that more women die of heart disease than of breast cancer and that hormones could prevent heart disease, few practitioners had the information to question this assumption. It became routine to prescribe hormones for heart disease prevention.

Let your practitioner know that you do not want to choose between heart disease and breast cancer! Now that research shows estrogen may not be effective against heart disease, it should be easier to discuss this issue with health care providers. There are many health-promoting ways to lower the risk of heart disease without increasing breast cancer risk.

The information on pages 46–50 summarizes what we know about the relationship between long-term use of estrogen and breast cancer and why mammography may be less effective in detecting early breast cancer in women on ERT or HRT. The woman who has a family history of pre-menopausal breast cancer, the woman who has already been on hormone products (i.e., women who were on high-dose birth control pills for many years), and any woman who is committed to minimizing her own breast cancer risk should be respected for questioning products whose long-term safety has not yet been established.

Some practitioners belittle women's worries about the breast cancer risks of hormones by explaining that if there is a risk, it is probably low. Breast cancer is the most prevalent cancer in women, so something that causes even a slight increase in risk affects many thousands of women. No woman wants to be one of those affected! Breast cancer is also a more common illness at young ages than heart disease, particularly for women who don't smoke.

Your provider validates your fear of breast cancer and encourages you to take one of the new wonder products (tamoxifen or raloxifene) to "prevent" breast cancer.

There is a huge difference between acknowledging that breast cancer is a major health issue for American women and taking health-promoting measures (low-fat diet, minimizing alcohol consumption, reducing intake of and exposure to carcinogenic chemicals) to reduce one's risk, and choosing to take new medications with serious side effects in hopes of reducing one's risk of breast cancer.

Pages 57–64 summarize the key issues about the new products being marketed for breast cancer prevention. While the long-term safety and the breast cancer prevention capabilities of these products have yet to be established, their manufacturers have carried out extremely effective advertising campaigns by playing on women's fears to promote their products. Similarly, your health practitioner has been bombarded with the drug companies' packaging of "the latest scientific findings" (from short-term studies) and may even be frightened into thinking that women could now sue their physicians if they are not offered "breast cancer prevention" drugs.

If you are interested in learning more about the new products, find someone who can work with you and realistically assess your breast cancer risk. In general, women's risk of being diagnosed with breast cancer has been exaggerated. Patricia Kelly's book, *Understanding Breast Cancer Risk* (Temple University Press, 1991), is recommended as a sensible guide. In addition, you can contact the National Women's Health Network Clearinghouse (202-628-7814 or www.womenshealthnetwork.org) to order a copy of our informational packet on breast cancer prevention.

You think you may want to take hormones.

Discuss why you may want to take hormones. Know that there is estrogen by itself (ERT) or estrogen plus progestin (HRT), both available in different brands and dosages and delivered in pills, patches, and creams. Expect your provider to take time to discuss which product will be best for you and why. Make certain that you remind your provider of any family history or other factors (such as whether or not you have a uterus) that you think affects your decision. Discuss the length of time you need to be taking hormones for the reason you are taking them (relatively short-term use for hot flashes or other specific symptoms;

longer use for osteoporosis prevention). You will also want to discuss how to maximize benefits of the treatment, such as exercise and dietary considerations, as well as arrange a follow-up visit. Reevaluate your decision periodically with someone you trust.

You are confused about whether to take hormones, but your provider is very strongly encouraging you to.

You do not have to make up your mind in the doctor's office! Ask the above set of questions, but know that taking a prescription home does not mean you immediately need to fill it. Once you do fill it, you can give yourself days or weeks to decide whether to start. Taking hormones is never a decision that has to be made immediately. Give yourself time to do more reading and discuss it with people you trust so that you feel good about whatever decision you eventually make.

If you decide to try HRT, do not second-guess your decision! Pay attention to how this medication suits you. (You may want to keep a journal before taking medication, and then while you are on hormones, see how you think it is affecting you.) If some day you decide to discontinue the prescription, make a plan with your health care provider to do it gradually, so that hot flashes or other menopausal symptoms are less likely to recur.

You have had a bone density screening test (at a women's health fair, at your workplace, in your clinic office) and someone has told you that you have low bone mass and should consider medication to prevent osteoporosis or because you already have osteoporosis.

Read chapter 10 to see how much debate there is over the definition of osteoporosis, what "low bone mass" means, and that bone mass screening of one part of your body does not necessarily predict what is happening elsewhere in your body. Don't be frightened into making a quick decision. Do know that making a plan to safely increase your weight-bearing exercise and getting sufficient calcium and vitamin D will be as important for strengthening your bones as your decision about medication.

If you decide that you are a candidate for medication, be sure to clarify exactly what the medication should do for you and how your health care provider plans to assess whether it is working. Currently, no products are approved for rebuilding bone. There are products that make BMD go up, but there is no evidence that fracture prevention is related to increasing bone density. Read the sections on hormones, SERMS, and new osteoporosis products and be aware that there are no long-term studies of any of the new osteoporosis products. You will want to follow the previous suggestions and pay particular attention to the question about how to take them, possible side effects, and getting regular checkups to make certain the medication suits you and serves its intended purpose.

You feel the need to urinate more frequently, even though your bladder isn't full, or your bladder leaks a little when you sneeze or laugh. Your health practitioner gives you a prescription for estrogen to remedy urinary incontinence.

Although estrogen is commonly prescribed for urinary incontinence, it has not been shown to be an effective treatment, and there is recent sound evidence that combination hormones actually make the situation worse. Read about how to do Kegel exercises on pages 234–235. Ask your practitioner about other ways to control urinary incontinence.

You have noticed lapses in your memory that trouble you, and your doctor suggests that taking estrogen might delay brain deterioration associated with aging.

Because of strongly held negative beliefs about aging in our culture, it is a challenge to enter your fifties enthusiastically. We tend to worry about details we associate with seemingly inevitable decline. Consequently, misplacing keys at age fifty-five takes on a more ominous tone than the same forgetful act at thirty-five. Although small studies have shown that estrogen does have physical effects on the brain, as yet there is not adequate evidence to support taking it to make our brains sharper. Read chapter 12 to get a more accurate view of aging, social conditions, and the ability to think and remember.

Until your mid-forties, you had monthly menses with three days moderate bleeding and two days lighter bleeding. For the past year, you have had menses about every three weeks with seven days of much heavier bleeding, often with large clots. After your period, you feel weaker, and walking your two miles three times a week for exercise seems much harder. You are visiting your nurse practitioner to discuss your concerns and options for treatment.

As you approach menopause, your ovaries may produce plenty of estrogen, but you probably will begin to skip ovulation and reduce production of progesterone. This results in thicker endometrial tissue and heavier blood loss during menstruation, which is very common during the perimenopausal years.

There can be other causes for this heavier bleeding— fibroids, for example—so you will want to request a pelvic exam and possibly a pelvic ultrasound to check for these conditions. Also, you will want to ask for a blood count (hemoglobin or hematocrit) to check for anemia. Whether or not you are diagnosed with anemia, you will want to make sure you are getting plenty of iron to replace the loss from heavy menstrual flow.

If other causes of heavy bleeding are ruled out, you have several options to alleviate this problem. Many women find that using lots of menstrual products (like wearing two pairs of underwear with thick pads in each!) and finding good friends to swap "heavy flow embarrassing moments" stories with is helpful to ease tension around this issue.

There are also medical options. Be reassured that this bleeding pattern will often resolve spontaneously as your ovaries decrease estrogen production, and any medical treatments usually last no longer than six to eighteen months. One option is adding oral progestin, either continuously or for about two weeks before your menses tend to start. Another option is low-dose birth control pills. Remember, these are needed only temporarily, and they do NOT obligate you to any longer term HRT use.

You had a few warm flushes for several months, but otherwise menopause was a breeze, and you have had no bleeding for eighteen months. You are delighted that menopause was so easy, but you now have moderately severe vaginal dryness that is uncomfortable during sexual activities. Your midwife, who delivered your daughter and your twin boys, recommends that you start HRT to treat the vaginal dryness.

There are many other solutions to this problem, and in fact, taking estrogen orally or using an estrogen patch sometimes does not relieve vaginal dryness effectively. Rather than systemic (affecting your whole body) hormone treatment, a first step can be the use of water-soluble lubricants during intercourse, bicycle riding, or other activities that are uncomfortable. You also can try vaginal estrogen creams, tablets, or a vaginal "estrogen ring" (left in place, it releases estrogen slowly and needs changing only every three months). These are low-dose estrogen solutions that may give you the benefit of lubrication without exposing you to risks associated with higher dosage oral or patch estrogens. For further discussion of these issues, see chapter 16.

You've heard that soy, herbs, or other alternative medicines may be good for menopause symptoms, but your health care provider dismisses those options or doesn't seem to know about them.

Most conventionally trained health care providers are not informed about alternative therapies. You can use the chapters of this book on phytoestrogens, natural hormones, and alternative approaches to inform yourself and share with your health care provider. If you're interested in pursuing such treatments, however, it's a good idea to find a health care provider who has experience working with them and—most important—is well-informed about what's known and not known about the risks and benefits of various options.

Your health care provider is an alternative medicine practitioner (naturopath, acupuncturist, herbalist, chiropractor, etc.) and has recommended that you take a dietary supplement, herb, or natural hormone product because you're approaching or experiencing menopause.

Many people don't realize that just as pharmaceutical companies promote drugs, so too is there a whole industry out there developing, producing, and selling dietary supplements, herbs, and other alternative health care products. Alternative health care practitioners are subject to similar influences from these companies as conventional doctors are from drug companies. These practitioners may promote a product they've seen in ads or have received free samples of from the manufacturer.

It's very important to know that herbs, natural hormones, and dietary supplements are not necessarily safe just because they're "natural." You will need to ask many of the same questions about alternative therapies as about a drug prescribed by a conventional doctor. Specifically, what is the reason to take it? Are there studies on this treatment showing that it is effective for the recommended purpose? What are the risks associated with it? An alternative product is less likely to have been studied, and you may decide to take it with less evidence of its efficacy than you would expect for a drug. But you will still want to learn what is known, consider any safety concerns, and be able to make an informed decision.

Reading the chapters of this book on phytoestrogens, herbs, natural hormones, and alternative approaches will give you reliable information about recommended alternative therapies for menopause symptoms. Some of them have long-established records of safe use for particular symptoms, while others are entirely unproven.

Don't leave your skepticism at the door just because you're seeing an alternative health care provider!

Most of all, try to find a knowledgeable health care provider who is willing to talk with you about your questions.

Notes

Introduction

   i. Calle EE, et al. Estrogen replacement therapy and risk of fatal colon cancer in a prospective cohort of postmenopausal women. *J Natl Cancer Inst* 87(7): 517–523, 1995.

  ii. Newcomb PA, Storer BE. Postmenopausal hormone use and risk of large-bowel cancer. *J Natl Cancer Inst* 87(14): 1067–1071, 1995.

 iii. Grodstein F, et al. Postmenopausal hormone use and risk for colorectal cancer and adenoma. *Ann Intern Med* 128(9): 705–712, 1998.

Chapter 1

1. Palmisano O, Edelstein J. Teaching drug promotion abuses to health profession students. *J Med Ed* 55: 453–455, 1980.

2. Ziegler MG, Lew P, Singer BC. The accuracy of drug information from pharmaceutical sales representatives. *JAMA* 273: 1296–1298, 1995.

3. Wilkes MS, Doblin BH, Shapiro MF. Pharmaceutical advertisements in leading medical journals: experts' assessments. *Ann Intern Med* 116: 912–919, 1992.

4. Rawlins MD. Doctors and the drug makers. *Lancet* 2: 276–278, 1984.

5. Bower AD, Burkett GL. Family physicians and generic drugs: a study of recognition, information sources, prescribing attitudes and practices. *J Fam Pract* 24(6): 612–616, 1987.

6. Caudill TS, Johnson MS, Rich EC, McKinney P. Physicians, pharmaceutical sales representatives, and the cost of prescribing. *Arch Fam Med* 5: 201–206, 1996.

7. Orentlicher D, Hehir MK II. Advertising policies of medical journals: conflicts of interest for journal editors and professional societies. *J Med Ethics* 27: 113–121, 1999.

8. Glassman P. Pharmaceutical advertising revenue and physician organizations: how much is too much? *West J Med* 171: 234–239, 1999.

9. Rochon PA, Gurwitz JH, Simms RW, et al. A study of manufacturer-supported trials of non-steroidal anti-inflammatory drugs in the treatment of arthritis. *Arch Intern Med* 154: 157–163, 1994.

10. Djulbegovic B, Lacevic M, Cantor A, et al. The uncertainty principle and industry-funded research. *Lancet* 356: 635–638, 2000.

11. Davidson RA. Source of funding and outcome of clinical trials. *J Gen Intern Med* 1: 155–158, 1986.

12. Stelfox HT, Chua G, O'Rourke K, Detsky AS. Conflict of interest in the debate over calcium channel antagonisters. *NEJM* 338: 101–105, 1998.

13. Friedberg M. Evaluation of conflict of interest in economic analyses of new drugs used in oncology. *JAMA* 282: 1453–1457, 1999.

14. Tarshis J. Celebrities reveal their secrets. *Parade* 14 March: 10–15, 2000.

15. Kolata G. Estrogen use tied to slight increase in risks to heart. *New York Times*, A1, 5 April 2000.

16. IMS Health. "IMS Health reports U.S. pharmaceutical promotional spending reached record $13.9 billion in 1999; direct-to-consumer spending up 40 percent year-over-year, to $1.8 billion." 20 April 2000.

17. *Prevention Magazine.* National survey of consumer reactions to direct-to-consumer advertising. Emmaus, PA: Rodale Press, 1998.

18. Bell RA, Wilkes MS, Kravitz RL. Advertisement-induced prescription drug requests: patients' anticipated reactions to a physician who refuses. *J Fam Pract* 48: 446–452, 1999.

19. Coalition of Labor Union Women, 1998.

20. Zones JS, Fugh-Berman A. Corporate funding and conflict of interest among U.S. non-profit women's health organizations. *Network News* May/June: 1–7, 1999.

21. Pooley J. Hamburger Helper for newscasters. *Brill's Content* December/January: 46, 1999.

22. Same as 21.

23. Moynihan R, et al. Coverage by the news media of the benefits and risks of medications. *NEJM* 342: 1645–1650, 2000.

24. *Hadassah.* Healthy women, healthy lives. http://www.hadassah.org/ WHealth/hwhl.htm. Accessed 2/9/01.

Chapter 2

1. Seaman B. *Women and the Crisis in Sex Hormones.* New York: Bantam Books, 1977.

2. Wilson RA. *Feminine Forever.* New York: Evans and Company, 1966, 132–133.

3. Clark P. Canada's foals. *ASPCA Animal Watch* Fall: 26–27, 1997.

4. Kennedy DL, et al. Non-contraceptive estrogens and progestins: use patterns over time. *Obstet Gynecol* 65(3): 441–446, 1985.

5. Smith DC, et al. Association of exogenous estrogen and endometrial carcinoma. *NEJM* 293(23): 1164–1167, 1975.

6. Ziel HK, Finkle WD. Increased risk of endometrial carcinoma among users of conjugated estrogens. *NEJM* 293(23): 1167–1170, 1975.

7. Ruzek SB. *The Women's Health Movement: Feminist Alternatives to Medical Control.* New York: Praeger, 1978.

8. Same as 4.

9. Grady D, et al. Hormone therapy to prevent disease and prolong life in postmenopausal women. *Ann Inern Med* 117(12): 1016–1037, 1992.

10. Same as 4.

11. Wysowski DK, et al. Use of menopausal estrogens and medroxyprogesterone in the United States, 1982–1992. *Obstet Gynecol* 85(1): 6–10, 1995.

12. Dejanikus T. Major drug manufacturer funds osteoporosis public education campaign. *Network News* 10(3): 1, 1985.

13. Consensus Conference. Osteoporosis. *JAMA* 252(6): 799–802, 1984.

14. Coney S. *The Menopause Industry: How the Medical Establishment Exploits Women.* Alameda, CA: Hunter House, 1994.

15. Same as 9.

16. U.S. Preventive Services Task Force. *Guide to Clinical Preventive Services*. Washington, D.C.: U.S. Government Printing Office, 1996.

17. Colditz GA, et al. Prospective study of estrogen replacement therapy and risk of breast cancer in postmenopausal women. *JAMA* 264(20): 2648–2653, 1990.

18. Steinberg KK, et al. A meta-analysis of the effect of estrogen replacement therapy on the risk of breast cancer. *JAMA* 265: 1985–1990, 1991.

19. Kolata G. Estrogen after menopause cuts heart attack risk, study finds. *New York Times* 12 September: A1, 1991.

20. Kolata G. Study links estrogen to cancer, but risk is slight. *New York Times* 28 November: A18, 1990.

21. Rinzler CA. *Estrogen and Breast Cancer: A Warning to Women*. New York: Macmillan, 1993.

22. Same as 14.

23. Fackelmann K. Forever smart. does estrogen enhance memory? *Science News* 147(5): 74–75, 1995.

24. Ruzek SB, Becker J. The women's health movement in the United States: from grassroots activism to professional agendas. *J Am Med Womens Assoc* 54(1): 4–8, 1999.

Chapter 3

1. Van Hall EV, Verdel M, Van der Velden J. "Perimenopausal" complaints in women and men: a comparative study. *J Womens Health* 3(1): 45–49, 1994.

2. Sloane E. *Biology of Women*. New York: John Wiley & Sons, 1993, 582–584.

3. Lock M. Contested meanings of menopause. *Lancet* 337: 1270–1272, 1991.

4. Beyene Y. Cultural significance and physiological manifestations of menopause. a biocultural analysis. *Cult Med Psychiatry* 10(1): 47–71, 1986.

5. Kaufert PA. The social and cultural context of menopause. *Maturitas* 23: 169–180, 1996.

6. McKinlay SM, et al. Women's experience of the menopause. *Curr Obstet Gynaecol* 1: 3–7, 1991.

7. Lock M. Menopause: lessons from anthropology. Presentation, North American Menopause Society, September 1995.

8. Porter M, et al. A population based survey of women's experience of the menopause. *Br J Obstet Gynaecol* 103: 1025–1028, 1996.

9. Seaman B. *Women and the Crisis in Sex Hormones*. New York: Bantam Books, 1977.

10. Andrews WC. The transitional years and beyond. *Obstet Gynecol* 85(1): 1–5, 1995.

11. Weiss KM. Evolutionary perspectives on human aging. In *Other Ways of Growing Old*, Amoss PT, Harrell S, eds. Stanford, CA: Stanford University Press, 1981: 25–28.

12. Lepine LA, et al. Hysterectomy surveillance—United States, 1980–1993. MMWR: *Morb Mortal Wkly Rep* 46(4): 1–5, 1997.

13. Colditz GA, et al. Menopause and the risk of coronary heart disease in women. *NEJM* 316(18): 1105–1110, 1987.

14. Wilcox LS, et al. Hysterectomy in the United States, 1988–1990. *Obstet Gynecol* 83(4): 549–555, 1994.

15. Langenberg G, et al. Hormone replacement and menopausal symptoms after hysterectomy. *Am J Epidemiol* 146(10): 870–880, 1997.

16. Cobb JO. *Understanding Menopause: Answers & Advice for Women in the Prime of Life*. New York: Penguin, 1988.

17. Wilcox LS, et al. Hysterectomy in the United States, 1988–1990. *Obstet Gynecol* 83(4): 549–555, 1994.

18. Same as 12.

19. Kerlikowske K, et al. Should women with familial ovarian cancer undergo prophylactic oophorectomy? *Obstet Gynecol* 80(4): 700–706, 1992.

20. Ford D, et al. Risks of cancer in BRCA1-mutation carriers. *Lancet* 343: 692–695, 1994.

21. Same as 19.

22. Runowicz CD. Advances in the screening and treatment of ovarian cancer. *Cancer J Clin* 42(6): 327-349, 1992.

23. Struewing JP, et al. Prophylactic oophorectomy in inherited breast/ovarian cancer families. *J Natl Cancer Inst Monogr* 17: 33–35, 1995.

24. Matloff ET, Shappell H, Brierly K, et al. What would you do? Specialists perspectives on cancer, genetic testing, prophylactic surgery and insurance discrimination. *J Clin Oncol* 18(12): 2484–2492, 2000.

25. Reichman BS, Green KB. Breast cancer in young women: effect of chemotherapy on ovarian function, fertility, and birth defects. *J Natl Cancer Inst Monogr* 16: 125–130, 1994.

26. Cobleigh ME, et al. Estrogen replacement therapy in breast cancer survivors: a time for change. *JAMA* 272(7): 540–545, 1994.

Chapter 4

1. Colditz GA. Relationship between estrogen levels, use of hormone replacement therapy, and breast cancer. *J Natl Cancer Inst* 90(11): 814–823, 1998.

2. Collaborative Group on Hormonal Factors in Breast Cancer. Breast cancer and hormone replacement therapy: collaborative reanalysis of data from 51 epidemiological studies of 52 705 women with breast cancer and 108 411 women without breast cancer. *Lancet* 350: 1047–1059, 1997.

3. Gambrell RD Jr. Hormone replacement therapy and breast cancer risk. *Arch Fam Med* 5(6): 341–348, 1996.

4. Grodstein F, Stampfer MJ, Colditz GA, et al. Postmenopausal hormone therapy and mortality. *NEJM* 336: 1769–1775, 1997.

5. Ettinger B, et al. Reduced mortality associated with long-term postmenopausal estrogen therapy. *Obstet Gynecol* 87(1): 6–12, 1996.

6. Willis DB, et al. Estrogen replacement therapy and risk of fatal breast cancer in a prospective cohort of postmenopausal women in the United States. *Cancer Causes Control* 7: 449–457, 1996.

7. Colditz GA, et al. The use of estrogens and progestins and the risk of breast cancer in postmenopausal women. *NEJM* 332: 1589–1593, 1995.

8. Bergkvist L, et al. The risk of breast cancer after estrogen and estrogen-progestin replacement. *NEJM* 321(5): 293–297, 1989.

9. Ewertz M, et al. Influence of non-contraceptive exogenous and endogenous sex hormones on breast cancer risk in Denmark. *Int J Cancer* 42: 832–838, 1988.

10. Ross RK, et al. Effect of hormone replacement therapy on breast cancer risk: estrogen versus estrogen plus progestin. *J Natl Cancer Inst* 92(4): 328–332, 2000.

11. Schairer C, et al. Menopausal estrogen and estrogen-progestin replacement therapy and breast cancer risk. *JAMA* 283(4): 485–491, 2000.

12. Laya MB, et al. Effect of postmenopausal hormone replacement therapy on mammographic density and parenchymal pattern. *Radiology* 196: 433–437, 1995.

13. Stomper PC, et al. Mammographic changes associated with post-menopausal hormone replacement therapy: a longitudinal study. *Radiology* 174: 487–490, 1990.

14. McNicholas MM, et al. Pain and increased mammographic density in women receiving hormone replacement therapy: a prospective study. *Am J Roentgenol* 163: 311–315, 1994.

15. Cohen MEL. Effect of hormone replacement therapy on cancer detection by mammography. *Lancet* 349: 1624, 1997.

16. Greendale GA, et al. Effects of estrogen and estrogen-progestin on mammographic parenchymal density. *Ann Intern Med* 130(4 Pt. 1): 262–269, 1999.

17. Laya MB. Effect of estrogen replacement therapy on the specificity and sensitivity of screening mammography. *J Natl Cancer Inst* 88(10): 643–649, 1996.

18. Grady D, et al. Hormone replacement therapy and endometrial cancer risk: a meta-analysis. *Obstet Gynecol* 85(2): 304–313, 1995.

19. The writing group for the PEPI trial. Effects of hormone replacement therapy on bone mineral density—results from the post-menopausal estrogen/progestin interventions (PEPI) trial. *JAMA* 276(17): 1389–1396, 1996.

20. Beresford SAA, et al. Risk of endometrial cancer in relation to use of oestrogen combined with cyclic therapy in postmenopausal women. *Lancet* 349: 458–461, 1997.

21. Pike MC, et al. Estrogen-progestin replacement therapy and endometrial cancer. *J Natl Cancer Inst* 89: 1110–1116, 1997.

22. Weiderpass E, Adami HO, Baron JA, Magnusson C, Bergstrom R, Lindgren A, Correia N, Persson I. Risks of endometrial cancer following estrogen replacement with and without progestins. *J Natl Cancer Inst* 91(13): 1131–1137, 1999.

23. Gruber DM, Wagner G, Kurz C, Sator MO, Huber JC. Endometrial cancer after combined hormone replacement therapy. *Maturitas* 31(3): 237–240, 1999.

24. Pike MC, Ross RK. Progestins and menopause: epidemiological studies of risks of endometrial and breast cancer. *Steroids* 65(10–11): 659–664, 2000.

25. Feeley KM, Wells M. Hormone replacement therapy and the endometrium. *J Clin Pathol* 54(6): 435–440, 2001.

26. Hill DA, Weiss NS, Beresford SA, Voigt LF, Daling JR, Stanford JL, Self S. Continuous combined hormone replacement therapy and risk of endometrial cancer. *Am J Obstet Gynecol* 183(6): 1456–1461, 2000.

27. Grady D, Ernster VL. Hormone replacement therapy and endometrial cancer: are current regimens safe? *J Natl Cancer Inst* 89(15): 1088–1089, 1997.

28. Garg PP, et al. Hormone replacement therapy and the risk of epithelial ovarian carcinoma: a meta-analysis. *Obstet Gynecol* 92(3): 472–479, 1998.

29. Prentice RL. On the epidemiology of oral contraceptives and disease. *Adv Cancer Res* 49: 285–401, 1987.

30. Thijs C, Knipschild P. Oral contraceptives and the risk of gallbladder disease: a meta-analysis. *Am J Public Health* 83(8): 1113–1120, 1993.

31. Petitti DB, et al. Increased risk of cholecystectomy in users of supplemental estrogen. *Gastroenterology* 94(1): 91–95, 1988.

32. Grodstein F, et al. Postmenopausal hormone use and cholecystectomy in a large prospective study. *Obstet Gynecol* 83(1): 5–11, 1994.

33. Ettinger B, et al. Gynecologic consequences of long-term unopposed estrogen replacement therapy. *Maturitas* 10: 271–282, 1988.

34. Ettinger B, et al. Gynecologic complications of cyclic estrogen progestin therapy. *Maturitas* 17: 197–204, 1993.

35. Daly E, et al. Risk of venous thromboembolism in users of hormone replacement therapy. *Lancet* 348: 977–980, 1996.

36. Jick H, et al. Risk of hospital admission for idiopathic venous thromboembolism among users of postmenopausal oestrogens. *Lancet* 348: 981–983, 1996.

37. Grodstein F, et al. Prospective study of exogenous hormones and risk of pulmonary embolism in women. *Lancet* 348: 983–987, 1996.

38. Grady D, et al. Postmenopausal hormone therapy increases risk for venous thromboembolic disease. the heart and estrogen/progestin replacement study. *Ann Intern Med* 132(9): 689–696, 2000.

39. Pedersen AT, et al. Hormone replacement therapy and risk of nonfatal stroke. *Lancet* 350: 1277–1283, 1997.

40. Petitti DB, et al. Ischemic stroke and the use of estrogen and estrogen/progestogen as hormone replacement therapy. *Stroke* 29(1): 23–28, 1998.

41. Grodstein F, et al. Postmenopausal hormone therapy and mortality. *NEJM* 336: 1769–1775, 1997.

42. Troisi RJ, et al. Menopause, postmenopausal estrogen preparations, and the risk of adult-onset asthma. *Am J Respir Crit Care Med* 152: 1183–1188, 1995.

43. Lieberman D, et al. Sub-clinical worsening of bronchial asthma during estrogen replacement therapy in asthmatic post-menopausal women. *Maturitas* 21: 153–157, 1995.

44. Sanchez-Guererro J, et al. Postmenopausal estrogen therapy and the risk for developing systemic lupus erythematosus. *Ann Intern Med* 122(6): 430–433, 1995.

45. Meier CR, et al. Postmenopausal estrogen replacement therapy and the risk of developing systemic lupus erythematosus or discoid lupus. *J Rheumatol* 25(8): 1515–1519, 1998.

Chapter 5

1. Fisher B, et al. Tamoxifen for prevention of breast cancer: report of the National Surgical Adjuvant Breast and Bowel Project P-1 Study. *J Natl Cancer Inst* 90(18): 1371–1389, 1998.

2. Gail MH, et al. Weighing the risks and benefits of tamoxifen treatment for preventing breast cancer. *J Natl Cancer Inst* 3 November: 1829–1846, 1999.

3. Delmas PD, et al. Effects of raloxifene on bone mineral density, serum cholesterol concentrations, and uterine endometrium in postmenopausal women. *NEJM* 337(23): 1641–1647, 1997.

4. Lufkin EG, et al. Treatment of established postmenopausal osteoporosis with raloxifene: a randomized trial. *J Bone Miner Res* 13(11): 1747–1754, 1998.

5. Ettinger B, et al. Reduction of vertebral fracture risk in postmenopausal women with osteoporosis treated with raloxifene. *JAMA* 282: 637–645, 1999.

6. Balfour JA, Goa KL. Raloxifene. *Drugs Aging* 12(4): 335–341, 1998.

7. Husten L. Raloxifene reduces breast-cancer risk. *Lancet* 353(9146): 44, 1999.

8. Barrett-Connor E, et al. Hormone and non-hormone therapy for the maintenance of postmenopausal health: the need for randomized controlled trials of estrogen and raloxifene. *J Womens Health* 7(7): 839–847, 1998.

9. Spencer CP, et al. Selective estrogen receptor modulators: women's panacea for the next millennium? *Am J Obstet Gynecol* 180(3 Pt 1): 763–770, 1999.

Chapter 6

1. Lock M. Contested meanings of menopause. *Lancet* 337(8752): 1270–1272, 1991.

2. Utian WH, Shoupe D, Bachmann G, et al. Relief of vasomotor symptoms and vaginal atrophy with lower doses of conjugated equine estrogens and medroxyprogesterone acetate. *Fertil Steril* 75: 1065–1079, 2001.

3. Baker VL. Alternatives to oral estrogen replacement. transdermal patches, percutaneous gels, vaginal creams and rings, implants, other methods of delivery. *Obstet Gynecol Clin North Am* 21(2): 271–297, 1994.

Chapter 7

1. Coward L, et al. Chemical modification of isoflavones in soy foods during cooking and processing. *Am J Clin Nutr* 68(6 Suppl): 1486S–1491S, 1998.

2. Thompson LU, Robb P, Serraino M, Cheung F. Mammalian lignan production from various foods. *Nutr Cancer* 16: 43–52, 1991.

3. Knight DC, Eden JA. A review of the clinical effect of phytoestrogens. *Obstet Gynecol* 87(5): 897–904, 1996.

4. Dalais FS, Rice GE, Wahlquist ML, Grehan M, Murkies AL, Medley G, Ayton R, Strauss BJG. Effects of dietary phytoestrogens in postmenopausal women. *Climacteric* 1: 124–129, 1998.

5. Adlercreutz H, Hamalainen E, Gorbach S, Goldin B. Dietary phytoestrogens and the menopause in Japan. *Lancet* 339: 1233, 1992.

6. Albertazzi P, Pansini F, Bonaccorsi G, et al. The effect of dietary soy supplementation on hot flushes. *Obstet Gynecol* 91: 6–11, 1998.

7. Brzezinski A, Adlercreutz H, Shaoul R, et al. Short-term effects of phytoestrogen-rich diet on postmenopausal women. *Menopause* 4(2): 89–94, 1997.

8. Murkies AL, Lombard C, Strauss BJG. Dietary flour supplementation decreases postmenopausal hot flushes: effect of soy and wheat. *Maturitas* 21: 189–195, 1995.

9. Dalais FS, Rice GE, Wahlquist ML, Grehan M, Murkies AL, Medley G, Ayton R, Strauss BJG. Effects of dietary phytoestrogens in postmenopausal women. *Climacteric* 1: 124–129, 1998.

10. Washburn S, Burke GL, Morgan T, Anthony M. Effect of soy protein supplementation on serum lipoproteins, blood pressure, and menopausal symptoms in perimenopausal women. *Menopause* 6: 7–13, 1999.

11. Wilcox G, Wahlqvist ML, Burger HG, Medley G. Oestrogenic effects of plant foods in postmenopausal women. *BMJ* 301: 905–906, 1990.

12. Baird DD, Umbach DM, Lansdell L, et al. Dietary intervention study to assess estrogenicity of dietary soy among postmenopausal women. *J Clin Endocrinol Metab* 80: 685–690, 1995.

13. Messina MJ, Persky V, Setchell KDR, Barnes S. Soy intake and cancer risk: a review of the in vitro and in vivo data. *Nutr Cancer* 21: 113–131, 1994.

14. Thompson LU, Robb P, Serraino M, Cheung F. Mammalian lignan production from various foods. *Nutr Cancer* 16: 43–52, 1991.

15. Lee H, Gourley L. Dietary effects on breast cancer in Singapore. *Lancet* 337: 1197–1200, 1991.

16. Yuan JM, Wang QS, Ross RK, et al. Diet and breast cancer in Shanghai and Tianjin, China. *Br J Cancer* 71: 1353–1358, 1995.

17. Ingram D, Sanders K, Kolybaba M, Lopez D. Case-control study of phyto-oestrogens and breast cancer. *Lancet* 350: 990–994, 1997.

18. Brzezinski A, Adlercreutz H, Shaoul R, et al. Short-term effects of phytoestrogen-rich diet on postmenopausal women. *Menopause* 4(2): 89–94, 1997.

19. Nomura A, Henderson B, Lee J. Breast cancer and diet among the Japanese in Hawaii. *Am J Clin Nutr* 31: 2020–2025, 1978.

20. Helferich WG. Paradoxical effects of the soy phytoestrogen, genistein on growth of human breast cancer cells in vitro and in vivo. Presented at Human Diet and Endocrine modulation: estrogenic and androgenic effects. International Life Sciences Institute of North America. Fairfax, VA, November 19–21, 1997.

21. Quella SK, et al. Evaluation of soy phytoestrogens for the treatment of hot flashes in breast cancer survivors: a North Central cancer treatment group trial. *J Clin Oncol* 18: 1068–1074, 2000.

22. Anderson JW, Johnstone BM, Cook-Newell ME. Meta-analysis of the effects of soy protein intake on serum lipids. *NEJM* 33: 276–282, 1995.

23. Clarkson TB, Anthony MS, Williams JK, et al. The potential for soybean phytoestrogens for postmenopausal hormone replacement therapy. *Proc Soc Exp Biol Med* 217: 365–368, 1998.

24. Goldberg J. Hip fracture incidence among elderly Asian-American populations. *Am J Epidemiol* 146(6): 502–509, 1997.

25. Cummings SR, Cauley JA, Palermo L, et al. Racial differences in hip axis length might explain racial differences in rates of hip fracture. Study of Osteoporotic Fractures Research Group. *Osteoporos Int* 4(4): 226–229, 1994.

26. Cooper C. The epidemiology of fragility fractures: is there a role for bone quality? *Calcif Tissue Int* 53(suppl 1): S23–S26, 1993.

27. Potter SM, Baum JA, Teng H, et al. Soy protein and isoflavones: their effects on blood lipids and bone density in postmenopausal women. *Am J Clin Nutr* 68(suppl): 1375S–1379S, 1998.

28. Alekal DL, et al. Isoflavone-rich soy protein isolate attenuates bone loss in the lumbar spine of perimenopausal women. *Am J Clin Nutr* 72(3): 844–852, 2000.

29. Arjmandi BH, Alekel L, Hollis BW, et al. Dietary soybean protein prevents bone loss in an ovariectomized rat model of osteoporosis. *J Nutr* 126: 161–167, 1996.

30. Fanti P, et al. The phytoestrogen genistein reduces bone loss in short-term ovariectomized rats. *Osteoporosis Intl* 8(3): 274–281, 1998.

31. Harrison E, et al. The effect of soybean protein on bone loss in a rat model of postmenopausal osteoporosis. *J Nutr Sci Vitaminol* (Tokyo) 44(2): 257–268, 1998.

32. Same as 30.

33. Fanti O, Faugere MC, Gang Z, et al. Systematic administration of genistein partially prevents bone loss in ovariectomized rats in a non-estrogen-like mechanism. *Am J Clin Nutr* 68(suppl): 1517S, 1998b.

34. Anderson JJ, Ambrose WW, Garner SC. Biphasic effects of genistein on bone tissue in the ovariectomized, lactating rat model. *Proc Soc Exp Biol Med* 217(3): 345–350, 1998.

35. Lees CJ, Ginn TA. Soy protein isolate diet does not prevent increased cortical bone turnover in ovariectomized macaques. *Calcif Tissue Int* 62(6): 557–558, 1998.

36. Same as 27.

37. Duke J. Beans to soy. *Alternative Therapies in Women's Health* 2(5): 36–38, 2000.

38. Kaufman PB, Duke JA, Brielmann H, Boik J, Hoyt JE. A comparative survey of leguminous plants as sources of the isoflavones genistein and daidzein: implications for human nutrition and health. *J Altern Complement Med* 3(1): 7–12, 1997.

39. Same as 38.

40. Anderson JW, Smith BM, Washnock CS. Cardiovascular and renal benefits of dry bean and soybean intake. *Am J Clin Nutr* 78(suppl): 464S–474S, 1999.

41. Knight DC, Eden JA. A review of the clinical effect of phytoestrogens. *Obstet Gynecol* 87(5): 897–904, 1996.

42. Setchell KDR. Phytoestrogens: the biochemistry, physiology and implications for human health of soy isoflavones. *Am J Clin Nutr* 68S: 133S–146S, 1998.

43. Goodman MT, Wilkems LR, Hankin JH, et al. Association of soy and fiber consumption with the risk of endometrial cancer. *Am J Epidemiol* 146: 294–306, 1997.

Chapter 8

1. Warnecke G. Beeinflussung klimakterischer Beschwerden durch ein Phytotherapeutikum: Erfolgreiche therapie mit Cimicifuga-Monoextrakt [Influence of phytotherapy on menopausal syndrome: successful treatments with monoextract of cimicifuga]. *Medizinische Welt* 36: 871–874, 1985.

2. Stoll W. Phytotherapeutikum beeinflusst atrophisches Vaginalepithel: Doppelblindversuch Cimicifuga vs. strogenpr parat [Phytotherapy influences atrophic vaginal epithelium—double-blind study—Cimicifuga vs. estrogenic substances]. *Therapeutikon* 1: 23–31, 1987.

3. Lehmann-Willenbrock E, Riedel H. Klinische und endokrinologische Untersuchengen zur Therapie ovarieller Ausfallserscheinungen nach Hysterektomie unter Belassung der Adnexe [Clinical and endocrinological examinations concerning therapy of climacteric symptoms following hysterectomy with remaining ovaries]. *Zentralbl Gynakol* 110: 611–618, 1988.

4. Same as 2.

5. Jacobson JS, et al. Randomized trial of black cohosh for the treatment of hot flashes among women with a history of breast cancer. *J Clin Oncol* 19(10): 2739–2745, 2001.

6. Same as 1.

7. Same as 2.

8. Same as 3.

9. Upton R, ed. Black Cohosh Rhizome. 2001 American Herbal Pharmacopoeia and Therapeutic Compendium, Santa Cruz, CA.

10. Fugh-Berman A, Awang D. Black cohosh. *Alternative Therapies in Womens Health* 3(11): 81–85, 2001.

11. Liu J, Burdette JE, Xu H, et al. Evaluation of estrogenic activity of plant extracts for the potential treatment of menopausal symptoms. *J Agric Food Chem* 49(5): 2472–2479, 2001.

12. Kruse SO, Lohning A, Pauli GF, Winterhoff H, Nahrstedt A. Fukiic and piscidic acid esters from the rhizome of Cimicifuga racemosa and the in vitro estrogenic activity of fukinolic acid. *Planta Med* 65(8): 763–764, 1999.

13. Jarry H, Harnischfeger G, Duker E. The endocrine effects of constituents of *Cimicifuga racemosa*. 2. In vitro binding of constituents to estrogen receptors. *Planta Med* 4: 316–319, 1985.

14. Struck D, Tegtmeier M, Harnischfeger G. Flavones in extracts of Cimicifuga racemosa. *Planta Med* 63: 289–290, 1997.

15. Hirata JD, et al. Does dong quai have estrogenic effects in post-menopausal women? A double-blind, placebo-controlled trial. *Fertil Steril* 68(6): 981–986, 1997.

16. Foster S, Tyler V. *Tyler's Honest Herbal,* 4th ed. New York: Haworth Press, 1999.

17. Fugh-Berman A. Herb-drug interactions. *Lancet* 355: 134–138, 2000.

18. Knight DC, Howes JB, Eden JA. The effect of Promensil, an isoflavone extract, on menopausal symptoms. *Climacteric* 2: 79–84, 1999.

19. Chenoy R, et al. Effect of oral gamolenic acid from evening primrose oil on menopausal flushing. *BMJ* 308: 501–503, 1995.

20. Fugh-Berman A, Cott J. Dietary supplements and natural products as psychotherapeutic agents. *Psychosom Med* 61: 712–728, 1999.

21. Oken BS, Storzbach DM, Kaye JA. The efficacy of Ginkgo biloba on cognitive function in Alzheimer disease. *Arch Neurol* 55(11): 1409–1415, 1998.

22. van Dongen MCJM, et al. The efficacy of ginkgo for elderly people with dementia and age-associated memory impairment: new results of a randomized clinical trial. *J Am Geriatr Soc* 48(10): 1183–1194, 2000.

23. Rai GS, et al. A double-blind, placebo-controlled study of Ginkgo biloba extract (Tanakan) in elderly outpatients with mild to moderate memory impairment. *Curr Med Res Opin* 12(6): 350–355, 1991.

24. Kleijnen J, Knipschild P. Ginkgo biloba for cerebral insufficiency. *Br J Clin Pharmacol* 34: 352–358, 1992.

25. Same as 18.

26. Wiklund IK, Mattsson LA, Lindgren R, et al. Effects of a standard-ized ginseng extract on quality of life and physiological parameters in symptomatic postmenopausal women: a double-blind, placebo-controlled trial. *Int J Clin Pharmacol Res* XIX(3): 89–99, 1999.

27. Punnonen R, Lukola A. Oestrogen-like effect of ginseng. *BMJ* 281: 1110, 1980.

28. Greenspan EM. Ginseng and vaginal bleeding. *JAMA* 249: 2018, 1983.

29. Hopkins MP, et al. Ginseng face cream and unexplained vaginal bleeding. *Am J Obstet Gynecol* 159: 1121–1122, 1988.

30. Palmer BV, et al. Ginseng and mastalgia. *BMJ* 1: 1284, 1978.

31. Koreich OM. Ginseng and mastalgia. *BMJ* 1: 1556, 1978.

32. Same as 17.

33. Same as 20.

34. Warnecke G, et al. Wirksamkeit von Kava-kava extrakt beim kli-makterischen syndrom. *Z Phytother* 11: 81–86, 1990.

35. Same as 35.

36. Same as 17.

37. Fugh-Berman A. *Alternative Medicine: What Works.* Baltimore: Lip-incott, Williams and Wilkins, 1997.

38. Same as 37.

39. Same as 16.

40. Barber RJ, Templeman C, Morton T, Kelley GE, West L. Random-ized placebo-controlled trial of an isoflavone supplement and menopausal symptoms in women. *Climacteric* 2: 85–92, 1999.

41. Same as 18.

42. Same as 40.

43. Same as 18.

44. Wichtl M. In *Herbal Drugs and Pharmaceuticals,* Bisset NM, ed. Stuttgart: Medpharm Scientific Publishers, 1994. Distributed by CRC Press, Boca Raton, FL.

45. Linde K, et al. St. John's Wort for depression—an overview and meta-analysis of randomized clinical trials. *BMJ* 313: 253–258, 1996.

Chapter 9

1. Regelson W, et al. Dehydroepiandrosterone (DHEA)—the "mother steroid." *Ann NY Acad Sci* 719: 553–563, 1994.

2. Beaulieu EE. Dehydroepiandrosterone (DHEA): a fountain of youth? *J Clin Endocrinol Metab* 81(9): 3147–3151, 1996.

3. Kroboth PD, et al. DHEA and DHEA-S: a review. *J Clin Pharmacol* 39(4): 327–348, 1999.

4. Morales AJ, et al. Effects of replacement dose of dehydroepiandrosterone in men and women of advancing age. *J Clin Endocrinol Metab* 78(6): 1360–1367, 1994.

5. Labrie F, et al. Effect of 12-month dehydroepiandrosterone replacement therapy on bone, vagina, and endometrium in postmenopausal women. *J Clin Endocrinol Metab* 82: 3498–3505, 1997.

6. Mitchell LE, et al. Evidence for an association between dehydroepiandrosterone sulfate and nonfatal, premature myocardial infarction in males. *Circulation* 89(1): 89–93, 1994.

7. Barrett-Connor E, et al. A prospective study of dehydroepiandrosterone sulfate, mortality and cardiovascular disease. *NEJM* 315: 1519–1524, 1986.

8. Barrett-Connor E, et al. Absence of an inverse relation of dehydroepiandrosterone sulfate with cardiovascular disease mortality in postmenopausal women. *NEJM* 317: 711, 1987.

9. Zumoff B, et al. Abnormal 24-hr mean plasma concentrations of dehydrepiandrosterone and dehydroepiandrosterone sulfate in women with primary operable breast cancer. *Cancer Res* 41: 3360–3363, 1981.

10. Helzsouer KJ, et al. Relationship of prediagnostic serum levels of dehydroepiandrosterone and dehydroepiandrosterone sulfate to the risk of developing premenopausal breast cancer. *Cancer Res* 52: 1–4, 1992.

11. Gordon GB, et al. Relationship of serum levels of dehydroepiandrosterone and dehydroepiandrosterone sulfate to the risk of developing postmenopausal breast cancer. *Cancer Res* 50: 3859–3862, 1990.

12. Dorgan JF. Relationship of serum dehydroepiandrosterone (DHEA), DHEA sulfate, and 5-androsterone-3 beta, 17 beta-diol to risk of breast cancer in postmenopausal women. *Cancer Epidemiol Biomarkers Prev* 6(3): 177–181, 1997.

13. Helzsouer KJ, et al. Serum gonadotropins and steroid hormones and the development of ovarian cancer. *JAMA* 274(24): 1926–1930, 1995.

14. LaBrie F, et al. Effect of 12-month dehydroepiandrosterone replacement therapy on bone, vagina, and endometrium in postmenopausal women. *J Clin Endocrinol Metab* 82(10): 3498–3505, 1997.

15. van Vollenhaven RF, et al. A double-blind, placebo-controlled, clinical trial of dehydroepiandrosterone in severe systemic lupus erythematosus. *Lupus* 8(3): 181–187, 1999.

16. Same as 14.

17. Morales AJ, et al. Effects of replacement dose of dehydroepiandrosterone in men and women of advancing age. *J Clin Endocrinol Metab* 78(6): 1360–1367, 1994.

18. Barnhart KT, et al. The effect of dehydroepiandrosterone supplementation to symptomatic perimenopausal women on serum endocrine profiles, lipid parameters, and health-related quality of life. *J Clin Endocrinol Metab* 84(11): 3896–3902, 1999.

19. Wolkowitz OM, et al. Double-blind treatment of major depression with dehydroepiandrosterone. *Am J Psychiatry* 156(4): 646–649, 1999.

20. Bloch M, et al. Dehydroepiandrosterone treatment of midlife dysthymia. *Biol Psychiatry* 45(12): 1533–1554, 1999.

21. Wolf OT, et al. Effects of a two-week physiological dehydroepiandrosterone substitution on cognitive performance and well-being in healthy elderly women and men. *J Clin Endocrinol Metab* 82(7): 2363–2367, 1997.

22. Wolf OT, et al. A single administration of dehydroepiandrosterone does not enhance memory performance in young healthy adults, but immediately reduces cortisol levels. *Biol Psychiatry* 42(9): 845–848, 1997.

23. Same as 17.

24. Vogiatzi MG, et al. Dehydroepiandrosterone in morbidly obese adolescents: effects on weight, body composition, lipids, and insulin resistance. *Metabolism* 45(8): 1011–1015, 1996.

25. Diamond P, et al. Metabolic effects of 12-month percutaneous dehydroepiandrosterone replacement therapy in postmenopausal women. *J Endocrinol* 150(suppl.): S43–S50, 1996.

26. Cardozo L, Bachmann G, McClish D, et al. Meta-analysis of estrogen therapy in the management of urogenital atrophy in postmenopausal women: second report of the Hormones and Urogenital Therapy Committee. *Obstet Gynecol* 92(4 Pt 2): 722–727, 1998.

27. Tzingounis VA, Aksu MF, Greenblatt RB. Estriol in the management of menopause. *JAMA* 239: 1638–1641, 1978.

28. Minaguchi H, Uemura T, Shirasu K, et al. Effect of estriol on bone loss in postmenopausal Japanese women: a multicenter prospective open study. *J Obstet Gynaecol Res* 22(3): 259–265, 1996.

29. Itoi H, Minakami H, Iwasaki R, Sato I. Comparison of the long-term effects of oral estriol with the effects of conjugated estrogen on serum lipid profile in early menopausal women. *Maturitas* 36(3): 271–222, 2000.

30. Lemon HM, Wotiz HH, Parsons L, Mozden PJ. Reduced estriol excretion in patients with breast cancer prior to endocrine therapy. *JAMA* 196: 112–120, 1966.

31. Lemon HM. Pathophysiologic considerations in the treatment of menopausal patients with oestrogens: the role of oestriol in the prevention of mammary carcinoma. *Acta Endocrinol* S233: 17–27, 1980.

32. Follingstad AH. Estriol, the forgotten estrogen? *JAMA* 239(1): 29–30, 1978.

33. Same as 32.

34. Lemon HM, Kumar PF, Peterson C, et al. Inhibition of radiogenic mammary carcinoma in rats by estriol or tamoxifen. *Cancer* 63(9): 1685–1692, 1989.

35. Same as 27.

36. Same as 32.

37. Lemon HM. Oestriol and prevention of breast cancer. *Lancet* 1(7802): 546–547, 1973.

38. Same as 27.

39. Van Haaften M, Donker GH, Sie-Go DM, et al. Biochemical and histological effects of vaginal estriol and estradiol applications on the endometrium, myometrium and vagina of postmenopausal women. *Gynecol Endocrinol* 11(3): 175–185, 1997.

40. Granberg S, Ylostalo P, Wikland M, Karlsson B. Endometrial sonographic and histologic findings in women with and without hormonal replacement therapy suffering from postmenopausal bleeding. *Maturitas* 27(1): 35–40, 1997.

41. Huether G. The contribution of extrapineal sites of melatonin synthesis to circulating melatonin levels in higher vertebrates. *Experientia* 79(8): 665–670, 1993.

42. Ekman AC, et al. Ethanol inhibits melatonin secretion in healthy volunteers in a dose-dependent randomized double-blind crossover study. *J Clin Endocrinol Metab* 77(3): 780–783, 1993.

43. Lee JR. *Natural Progesterone: The Multiple Roles of a Remarkable Hormone*. Sepastopol, CA: BLL Publishing, 1993.

44. Lee JR. Osteoporosis reversal with transdermal progesterone. *Lancet* 336: 1327, 1990.

45. Leonetti HB, Longo S, Anasti JN. Transdermal progesterone cream for vasomotor symptoms and postmenopausal bone loss. *Obstet Gynecol* 94: 225–228, 1999.

46. King RJB. A discussion of the roles of oestrogen and progestin in human mammary corcinogenesis. *J Steroid Biochem Mol Biol* 39: 811–818, 1991.

47. Staffa JA, et al. Progestins and breast cancer: an epidemiological review. *Fertil Steril* 57: 473–491, 1992.

48. Schairer C, et al. Menopausal estrogen and estrogen-progestin replacement therapy and breast cancer risk. *JAMA* 283(4): 485–491, 2000.

49. Nason FG, Nelson BE. Estrogen and progesterone in breast and gynecological cancers. *Obstet Gynecol Clin North Am* 21: 245–270, 1994.

50. Cooper A, Spencer C, Whitehead MI, et al. Systemic absorption of progesterone from Progest cream in postmenopausal women. *Lancet* 351: 1255–1256, 1998.

51. MacFarland SA. Use of Pro-Gest cream in postmenopausal women. *Lancet* 352: 905, 1998.

52. Lee JR. Use of Pro-Gest cream in postmenopausal women. *Lancet* 352: 905, 1998.

53. Passeri M, Biondi M, Costi D, et al. Effects of 2-year ipriflavone in elderly women with established osteoporosis. *Ital J Miner Electrolyte Metab* 9: 136–144, 1995.

54. Agnusdei D, Bufalino L. Efficacy of ipriflavone in established osteoporosis and long-term safety. *Calcif Tissue Int* 61: S23–S27, 1997.

55. Maugeri D, Panebianco P, Russo MS, et al. Ipriflavone treatment of senile osteoporosis: results of a multicenter, double-blind clinical trial of 2 years. *Arch Gerentol Geriatr* 19: 253–263, 1994.

56. Adami S, Bufalino L, Cervetti R, et al. Ipriflavone prevents radial bone loss in postmenopausal women with low bone mass over 2 years. *Osteoporos Int* 7: 119–125, 1997.

57. Gennari C, Adami S, Agnusdei D, et al. Effect of chronic treatment with ipriflavone in postmenopausal women with low bone mass. *Calcif Tissue Int* 61: S19–S22, 1997.

58. Gennari C, Agnusdei D, Crepaldi G, et al. Effect of ipriflavone—a synthetic derivative of natural isoflavones—on bone mass loss in the early years after menopause. *Menopause* 5(1): 9–15, 1998.

59. Ohta H, Komukai S, Makita K, et al. Effects of 1-year ipriflavone treatment on lumbar bone mineral density and bone metabolic markers in postmenopausal women with low bone mass. *Horm Res* 51(4): 178–183, 1999.

60. Valente M, Bufalino L, Casiglione GN, et al. Effects of 1-year treatment with ipriflavone on bone in postmenopausal women with low bone mass. *Calcif Tissue Int* 54(5): 377–380, 1994.

61. Nozaki M, Hashimoto K, Inoue Y, et al. Treatment of bone loss in oophorectomized women with a combination of ipriflavone and conjugated equine estrogen. *Int J Gynecol Obstet* 62(1): 69–75, 1998.

62. De Aloysio D, Gambacciani M, Altieri P. Bone density changes in postmenopausal women with the administration of ipriflavone alone or in association with low-dose ERT. *Gynecol Endocrinol* 11: 289–293, 1997.

63. Gambacciani M, Ciaponi M, Cappagli B, et al. Effects of combined low dose of the isoflavone derivative ipriflavone and estrogen replacement on bone mineral density and metabolism in post-menopausal women. *Maturitas* 28(1): 75–81, 1997.

64. Ibid.

65. Cecchettin M, Bellometti S, Cremonesi G, et al. Metabolic and bone effects after administration of ipriflavone and salmon calcitonin in postmenopausal osteoporosis. *Biomed Pharmacother* 49(10): 465–468, 1995.

Chapter 10

1. Looker AC, et al. Prevalence of low femoral bone density in older US women from NHANES III. *J Bone Miner Res* 10(5): 796–802, 1995.

2. Melton LJ, et al. How many women have osteoporosis? *J Bone Miner Res* 7(9): 1005–1010, 1992.

3. Chrischilles EA, et al. A model of lifetime osteoporosis impact. *Arch Intern Med* 151: 2026–2032, 1991.

4. Cummings SR, et al. Should prescription of postmenopausal hormone therapy be based on the results of bone densiometry? *Ann Intern Med* 113(8): 565–567, 1990.

5. Jacobsen SJ, et al. Race and sex differences in mortality following fracture of the hip. *Am J Public Health* 82(8): 1147–1150, 1992.

6. Boodman SG. Hard evidence. *Washington Post Health Magazine,* September 26, 2000.

7. Same as 6.

8. Nieves JW, et al. Calcium potentiates the effect of estrogen and calcitonin on bone mass: review and analysis. *Am J Clin Nutr* 67(1): 18–24, 1998.

9. Ettinger B. Update: estrogen and postmenopausal osteoporosis. *Health Values* 11(4): 31–36, 1987.

10. Lock M. Contested meanings of menopause. *Lancet* 337(8752): 1270–1272, 1991.

11. Report of a WHO study group. Assessment of fracture risk and its application to screening for postmenopausal osteoporosis. WHO technical report series: 843, 1994.

12. Same as 2.

13. Riggs BL, Melton LJ. Involutional osteoporosis. *NEJM* 314(26): 1676–1686, 1986.

14. Albala C, et al. Obesity as a protective factor for postmenopausal osteoporosis. *Int J Obes* 20: 1027–1032, 1996.

15. Rosen CJ, et al. Elderly women in northern New England exhibit seasonal changes in bone mineral density and calciotrophic hormones. *Bone Miner* 25: 83–92, 1994. Cited in Kardinaal AFM, et al. Dietary calcium and bone density in adolescent girls and young women in Europe. *J Bone Miner Res* 14(4): 583–592, 1999.

16. McClung MR, Goldstein SR. Potential impact of emerging therapies on osteoporosis prevention (symposium presentation). Reported in *Am J Managed Care* 4(2 suppl): S78–S84, 1998.

17. Ringa V, et al. Bone mass measurements around menopause and prevention of osteoporotic fractures. *Eur J Obstet Gynecol Reprod Biol* 54: 205–213, 1994.

18. An emerging approach to osteoporosis prevention. Discussion at Clinical and Economic Considerations in the Prevention of Osteoporosis Among Postmenopausal Women Conference, September 19, 1997. Reported in *Am J Managed Care* 4(2 suppl): S85–S93, 1998.

19. Marshall D, et al. Meta-analysis of how well measures of bone density predict occurrence of osteoporotic fractures. *BMJ* 312: 1254–1259, 1996.

20. Anonymous. FDA Committee wary on surrogate markers in osteoporosis trials. Script no. 1719: 21, May 20, 1992. Cited by Kanis J. Treatment of osteoporosis in elderly women. *Am J Med* 98(2A): 2A–60S, 1995.

21. National Institutes of Health Consensus Development Conference Statement. Osteoporosis prevention, diagnosis and therapy. March 27–29, 2000.

22. British Columbia Office of Health Technology Assessment. Bone mineral density testing: does the evidence support its selective use in well women. December, 1997. BCOHTA 97: 2T publication.

23. Kiel DP, et al. Hip fracture and the use of estrogens in postmenopausal women. *NEJM* 317(19): 1169–1174, 1987.

24. Riis BJ, et al. The effect of percutaneous estradiol and natural progesterone on postmenopausal bone loss. *Am J Obstet Gynecol* 156(1): 61–65, 1987.

25. Christiansen C, et al. Five years with continuous combined oestrogen/progestogen therapy. Effects on calcium metabolism, lipoproteins, and bleeding pattern. *Br J Obstet Gynaecol* 97: 1087–1092, 1990.

26. Marslew U, et al. Two new combinations of estrogen and progestogen for prevention of postmenopausal bone loss: long-term effects on bone. *Obstet Gynecol* 79(2): 202–210, 1992.

27. The writing group for the PEPI trial. Effects of hormone replacement therapy on bone mineral density—results from the postmenopausal estrogen/progestin interventions (PEPI) trial. *JAMA* 276(17): 1389–1396, 1996.

28. Naessen T, et al. Hormone replacement therapy and the risk for first hip fracture. *Ann Intern Med* 113(2): 95–103, 1990.

29. Cauley JA, et al. Estrogen replacement therapy and fractures in older women. *Ann Intern Med* 122(1): 9–16, 1995.

30. Assessment of fracture risk and its application to screening for postmenopausal osteoporosis. WHO Technical Report Series 843. Geneva: WHO, 1994. Cited by Kanis J. Treatment of osteoporosis in elderly women. *Am J Med* 98(2A): 2A–60S, 1995.

31. Genant HK, et al., for the Estratab-Osteoporosis Study Group. Low dose esterified estrogen therapy. *Arch Intern Med* 157: 2609–2615, 1997.

32. Libanati C. Prevention and treatment of osteoporosis. *Prim Care Rep* 5(5): 27–34, 1999.

33. Rosenberg S, et al. Decrease of bone mineral density during estrogen substitution therapy. *Maturitas* 17(3): 205–210, 1993.

34. Aitken JM, et al. Oestrogen replacement therapy for prevention of osteoporosis after oophorectomy. *BMJ* (3): 515–518, 1973.

35. Ensrud KE, et al. Hip bone loss increases with advancing age: longitudinal results from the study of osteoporotic fractures. Raisz LG, ed. Sixteenth Annual Meeting of the American Society for Bone and Mineral Research. Kansas City, MO: Mary Ann Liebert, 1994, S153. Cited in Black DM. Why elderly women should be screened and treated to prevent osteoporosis. *Am J Med* 98(2A): 67S–75S, 1995.

36. Black DM. Why elderly women should be screened and treated to prevent osteoporosis. *Am J Med* 98(2A): 67S–75S, 1995.

37. Same as 29.

38. Felson DT, et al. The effect of postmenopausal therapy on bone density in elderly women. *NEJM* 329: 1141–1146, 1993.

39. Ettinger B, Grady D. The waning effect of postmenopausal estrogen therapy on osteoporosis. *NEJM* 329(16): 1192–1193, 1993.

40. Steinberg KK, et al. A meta-analysis of the effect of estrogen replacement therapy on the risk of breast cancer. *JAMA* 265(15): 1985–1990, 1991.

41. Schneider DL, et al. Timing of postmenopausal estrogen for optimal bone mineral density. *JAMA* 277(7): 543–547, 1997.

42. Michaelsson K, et al. Hormone replacement therapy and the risk of hip fracture: population based case control study. *BMJ* 316: 1858–1862, 1998.

43. Same as 36.

44. Notelovitz M, Ware M. Presented at September 1996 North American Menopause Society Annual Meeting. Reported in Notebook, *J Womens Health* 5: 537, 1996.

45. Ettinger B, et al. Postmenopausal bone loss is prevented by treatment with low-dosage estrogen with calcium. *Ann Intern Med* 106: 40–45, 1987.

46. Ettinger B. Use of low-dose 17 beta-estradiol for the prevention of osteoporosis. *Clin Ther* 15(6): 950–962, 1993.

47. Associated Press. Lower estrogen dosage OKd for osteoporosis. *San Francisco Chronicle* March 12, A7, 1998.

48. Same as 31.

49. Naessen T, et al. Bone loss in elderly women prevented by ultra-low doses of parenteral 17B-estradiol. *Am J Obstet Gynecol* 177(1): 115–119, 1997.

50. Cummings SR, et al., for the Study of Osteoporotic Fractures Research Group. Endogenous hormones and the risk of hip and vertebral fractures among older women. *NEJM* 339(11): 733–738, 1998.

51. Raisz L, Prestwood KM. Estrogen and the risk of fracture—new data, new questions. *NEJM* 339(11): 767–768, 1998.

52. Lucas GH, et al. Low-dose esterified estrogen therapy. Effects on bone, plasma estradiol concentrations, endometrium and lipid levels. *Arch Intern Med* 157: 2609–2615, 1997. Cited in Freeman R. The management of the patient with osteoporosis—a modern epidemic. *Am J Managed Care* 4(2 suppl): S94–S107, 1998.

53. Wallach S. Osteoporosis treatment regimens: past, present, future. *Menopause Management* II(4): 14, 1993.

54. McClung MR, Goldstein SR. "Potential impact of emerging therapies on osteoporosis prevention," symposium presentation. Reported in *Am J Managed Care* 4(2 suppl): S78–S84, 1998.

55. Same as 27.

56. Lyritis GP, et al. Analgesic effect of salmon calcitonin in osteoporotic vertebral fracture: a double-blind placebo-controlled study. *Calcif Tissue Int* 49: 369–372, 1991. Cited in Libanati C. Prevention and treatment of osteoporosis. *Prim Care Rep* 5(5): 27–34, 1999.

57. The Medical Letter. Report on osteoporosis products. January 5. Cited in *HealthFacts* (Center for Medical Consumers) 21(201): 3–4, 1996.

58. Freeman R. The management of the patient with osteoporosis—a modern epidemic. *Am J Managed Care* 4(2 suppl): S94–S107, 1998.

59. Black DM, et al. Randomized trial of effect of alendronate on risk of fracture in women with existing vertebral fractures. *Lancet* 348: 1535–1541, 1996.

60. Hosking D, et al. Prevention of bone loss with alendronate in postmenopausal women under 60 years of age. *NEJM* 338(8): 485–492, 1998.

61. Ensrud KE, et al., for the Fracture Intervention Trial Research Group. Treatment with alendronate prevents fractures in women at highest risk. *Arch Intern Med* 157: 2617–2624, 1997.

62. Cummings SR, et al., for the Fracture Intervention Trial Research Group. Effect of alendronate on risk of fracture in women with low bone density but without vertebral fractures. *JAMA* 280(24): 2077–2082, 1998.

63. Gharib SD. Alendronate lowers fracture risk. *Journal Watch—Women's Health* 4(2): 9, 1999.

64. Same as 62.

65. Same as 63.

66. Heaney RD. Bone mass, bone fragility, and the decision to treat. *JAMA* 28(24): 2119–2120, 1998.

67. Same as 62.

68. Same as 63.

69. Tanouye E. Merck's osteoporosis warnings pave the way for its new drug. *Wall Street Journal*, June 28, 1995.

70. Annual Adverse Drug Experience Report, 1996, http://www.fda.gov/cder/dpe/annrep96/index.htm.

71. Sherwood L. Presentation to FDA Radiological Devices Panel meeting, May 17, 1999.

72. Raymond SC. Letter to Cynthia A. Pearson, January 15, 1999.

73. Reb AM (Regulatory Review Officer). Correspondence from the Division of Drug Marketing, Advertising and Communications, Food and Drug Administration dated April 14, 1997, and July 2, 1997, to Ellen R. Westrick, Senior Director, Office of Medical/Legal Issues, Merck.

74. Same as 63.

75. Libanati C. Prevention and treatment of osteoporosis. *Prim Care Rep* 5(5): 27–34, 1999.

76. Graham D, Malaty HM, Goodgame R. Primary amino-bisphosphonates: a new class of gastrotoxic drugs—comparison of alendronate and aspirin. *Am J Gastroenterol* 92(8): 1322–1325, 1997.

77. Graham DY. Excess gastric ulcers are associated with alendronate therapy. *Am J Gastroenterol* 93(8): 1395, 1998.

78. Ettinger B, et al. Alendronate use among 812 women: prevalence of gastrointestinal complaints, noncompliance with patient instructions and discontinuation. *J Managed Care Phar* 4(5): 488–492, 1998.

79. Same as 63.

80. Same as 75.

81. Same as 77.

82. Same as 77.

83. Ettinger B, Pressman A, Schein J. Clinic visits and hospital admissions for care of acid-related upper gastrointestinal disorders in women using alendronate for osteoporosis. *Am J Managed Care* 4(10): 1377–1382, 1998.

84. Pearson C. Alendronate for osteoporosis. National Women's Health Network testimony before the FDA Endocrinologic and Metabolic Drugs Advisory Committee, July 13, 1995.

85. Cadogan J, et al. Milk intake and bone mineral acquisition in adolescent girls: randomized, controlled intervention trial. *BMJ* 315: 1255–1260, 1997.

86. Silverman SL, et al. Effect of bone density information on decisions about hormone replacement therapy: a randomized trial. *Obstet Gynecol* 89: 321–325, 1997. Referred to in Lindsay R, et al. Current approaches to osteoporosis prevention, symposium presentation. *Am J Managed Care* 4(2 suppl.): S64–S69, 1998.

87. Silverman SL, et al. Effect of bone density information on decisions about hormone replacement therapy: a randomized trial. *Obstet Gynecol* 89: 321–325, 1997. Referred to in Lindsay R, et al. Current approaches to osteoporosis prevention (symposium presentation). *Am J Managed Care* 4(2 suppl): S64–S69, 1998.

88. Torgerson DJ, et al. Randomized trial of osteoporosis screening: use of hormone replacement therapy and quality of life results. *Arch Intern Med* 157: 2121–2125, 1997.

89. Freeman R. The management of the patient with osteoporosis—a modern epidemic. *Am J Managed Care* 4(2 suppl): S94–S107, 1998.

90. Dawson-Hughes B. The role of calcium in the prevention and treatment of osteoporosis. Abstract of presentation at NIH Consensus Development Conference on Osteoporosis Prevention, Diagnosis, and Therapy, 2000.

91. Rubin SM, Cummings SR. Results of bone densitometry affect women's decisions about taking measures to prevent fractures. *Ann Intern Med* 116(12 pt 1): 990–995, 1992.

92. Cauley J, et al. Bone mineral density and risk of breast cancer in older women. *JAMA* 276(17): 1404–1408, 1996.

93. Lucas FL, et al., for the Osteoporotic Fracture Research Group. Bone mineral density and risk of breast cancer—differences by family history of breast cancer. *Am J Epidemiol* 148(1): 22–29, 1998.

Chapter 11

1. Speroff L. From OCs to replacement therapy: a strategy for transition. *Dialogues in Contraception* 2(8): 1–6, 1989.

2. Bush T. Feminine forever revisited: menopausal hormone therapy in the 1990s. *J Womens Health* 1(1): 1–4, 1992.

3. Egeland G. Characteristics of noncontraceptive hormone users. *Prev Med* 17: 403–411, 1988.

4. Posthuma WFW, et al. Cardioprotective effect of hormone replacement therapy in postmenopausal women: is the evidence biased? *BMJ* 308: 1268–1269, 1994.

5. Barrett-Connor E. Postmenopausal estrogen and prevention bias. *Ann Intern Med* 115(6): 455–456, 1991.

6. Kritz-Silverstein D, et al. Long-term postmenopausal hormone use, obesity, and fat distribution in older women. *JAMA* 275(1): 46–49, 1996.

7. Hemminki E, Sihvo S. A review of postmenopausal hormone therapy recommendations: potential for selection bias. *Obstet Gynecol* 82: 1021–1028, 1993.

8. Birnbaum D, Pearson C. Proposed cardiovascular indication for Premarin (presentation). FDA Fertility and Maternal Health Drugs Advisory Committee meeting, June 14–15, 1990.

9. Hulley S, et al. Randomized trial of estrogen plus progestin for secondary prevention of coronary heart disease in postmenopausal women. *JAMA* 280(7): 605–613, 1998.

10. Lenfant C. Statement from Claude Lenfant, MD, NHLBI director, on preliminary trends in the women's health initiative. *NIH Backgrounder*, April 3, 2000.

11. Kolata G. Estrogen use tied to slight increase in risks to heart. *New York Times*, 5 April: A1, 2000.

12. Grodstein F, et al. Postmenopausal hormone therapy and mortality. *NEJM* 336: 1769–1775, 1997.

13. Petitti DB. Coronary heart disease and estrogen replacement therapy: can compliance bias explain the results of observational studies? *Ann Epidemiol* 4: 115–118, 1994.

14. The Coronary Drug Project Research Group. Influence of adherence to treatment and the response of cholesterol mortality in the Coronary Drug Project. *NEJM* 303: 1033–1041, 1980.

15. Horwitz RI, Viscoli CM, Berkman L, et al. Treatment adherence and risk of death after a myocardial infarction. *Lancet* 336: 542–545, 1990.

16. Same as 10.

17. Hulley S, et al. Randomized trial of estrogen plus progestin for secondary prevention of coronary heart disease in postmenopausal women. *JAMA* 280(7): 605–613, 1998.

18. Herrington DM, et al. Effects of estrogen replacement on the progression of coronary-artery atherosclerosis. *NEJM* 343(8): 572–574, 2000.

19. Cauley JA, et al. Estrogen replacement therapy and mortality among older women. The study of osteoporotic fractures. *Arch Intern Med* 157(19): 2181–2187, 1997.

20. Heckbert SR, et al. Duration of estrogen replacement therapy in relation to the risk of incident myocardial infarction in postmenopausal women. *Arch Intern Med* 157(12): 1330–1336, 1997.

21. Stampfer MJ, et al. Postmenopausal estrogen therapy and cardiovascular disease. *NEJM* 325(11): 756–762, 1991.

22. Sidney S, et al. Myocardial infarction and the use of estrogen and estrogen-progestogen in postmenopausal women. *Ann Intern Med* 127: 501–508, 1997.

23. McLaughlin VV, et al. Relation between hormone replacement therapy in women and coronary artery disease estimated by electron beam tomography. *Am Heart J* 134(6): 1115–1119, 1997.

24. Hemminki E, McPherson K. Impact of postmenopausal hormone therapy on cardiovascular events and cancer: pooled data from clinical trials. *BMJ* 315: 149–153, 1997.

25. Wysowski DK, et al. Use of menopausal estrogens and medroxyprogesterone in the United States, 1982–1992. *Obstet Gynecol* 85(1): 6–10, 1995.

26. Barrett-Connor E, Corady D. Hormone replacement therapy, heart disease, and other considerations. *Ann Rev Public Health* 128(9): 705–712, 1998.

27. Grodstein F, et al. Postmenopausal estrogen and progestin use and the risk of cardiovascular disease. *NEJM* 335(7): 453–461, 1996.

28. The writing group for the PEPI trial. Effects of estrogen or estrogen/progestin regimens on heart disease risk factors in postmenopausal women. *JAMA* 273(3): 199–208, 1995.

29. Miyagawa K, et al. Medroxyprogesterone interferes with ovarian steroid protection against coronary vasospasm. *Nat Med* 3: 324–327, 1997.

30. Raloff J. Hormone therapy: issues of the heart. *Science News* 151: 40, 1997.

31. US Mortality Tapes. National Center for Health Statistics. US Dept of Health and Human Services (DHHS), Hyattsville, MD, 1968–1983.

32. Tunstall-Pedoe H. Myth and paradox of coronary risk and the menopause. *Lancet* 351: 1425–1427, 1998.

33. MacPherson KI. Cardiovascular disease in women and noncontraceptive use of hormones: a feminist analysis. *Adv Nursing Sci* 14(4): 34–49, 1992.

34. Doress PD, Siegal DL. *Ourselves, Growing Older*. New York: Simon and Schuster, 1994.

35. Stampfer M. Proposed cardioprotective indication for Premarin (presentation). FDA Fertility and Maternal Health Drugs Advisory Committee meeting, June 15, 1990, transcript page 47.

36. Toosz-Hobson P, et al. Hormone replacement therapy for all? Universal prescription is desirable. *BMJ* 313(7053): 350–351, 1996.

Chapter 12

1. Ernst RL, Hay JW. The U.S. economic and social costs of Alzheimer's disease revisited. *Am J Public Health* 262: 2551–2556, 1994.

2. Burns A, Murphy D. Protection against Alzheimer's disease? *Lancet* 348: 420–421, 1996.

3. Wickelgren I. Estrogen stakes claim to cognition. *Science* 276: 675–678, 1997.

4. Yaffe K, et al. Estrogen therapy in postmenopausal women—effects on cognitive function and dementia. *JAMA* 279(9): 688–695, 1998.

5. Barrett-Connor E. Rethinking estrogen and the brain. *J Am Geriatr Soc* 46: 918–920, 1998.

6. Shaywitz SE, et al. Effect of estrogen on brain activation patterns in postmenopausal women during working memory tasks. *JAMA* 281(13): 1197–1202, 1999.

7. Gould E, et al. Neurogenesis in the neocortex of adult primates. *Science* 286: 548–552, 1999.

8. Baldereschi M, et al. Estrogen-replacement therapy and Alzheimer's disease in the Italian Longitudinal Study on Aging. *Neurology* 50: 996–1002, 1998.

9. Jacobs D, et al. Cognitive function in nondemented older women who took estrogen after menopause. *Neurology* 50: 368–373, 1998.

10. Waring S, et al. Postmenopausal estrogen replacement therapy and risk of AD—a population-based study. *Neurology* 52: 965–970, 1999.

11. Same as 10.

12. Yaffe K, Grady D, Pressman A, Cummings S. Serum estrogen levels, cognitive performance, and risk of cognitive decline in older community women. *J Am Geriatr Soc* 46: 816–821, 1998.

13. Polo-Kantola P, et al. The effect of short-term estrogen replacement therapy on cognition: a randomized, double-blind, cross-over trial in postmenopausal women. *Obstet Gynecol* 91: 459–466, 1998.

14. Greendale GA, et al. Symptom relief and side effects of postmenopausal hormones: results from the Postmenopausal Estrogen/Progestin Intervention trial. *Obstet Gynecol* 92: 982–988, 1998.

15. Greenough WT, Cohen NJ, Juraska JM. New neurons in old brains: learning to survive? *Nat Neurosci* 2(3): 203–205, 1999.

16. Diamond MC. *Enriching Heredity: The Impact of the Environment on the Anatomy of the Brain.* New York: Free Press, 1988.

17. White L, et al. Prevalence of dementia in older Japanese-American men in Hawaii—The Honolulu-Asian Aging Study. *JAMA* 276(12f): 955–960, 1996.

18. Jean H, et al. Alzheimer's disease: preliminary study of spatial distribution at birth place. *Soc Sci Med* 42(6): 871–878, 1996.

19. Same as 10.

20. Same as 9.

21. Callahan C, et al. Relationships of age, education, and occupation with dementia among a community-based sample of African-Americans. *Arch Neurol* 53: 134–140, 1996.

22. Bassuk SS, et al. Social disengagement and incident cognitive decline in community-dwelling elderly persons. *Ann Intern Med* 131(3): 165–173, 1999.

23. Maisie HE. Linguistic ability in early life and Alzheimer's disease in late life. Letter. *JAMA* 275(24): 1879, 1996.

24. Snowdon DA, et al. Linguistic ability in early life and cognitive function and Alzheimer's disease in late life. *JAMA* 275(7): 528–532, 1996.

25. Muntaner C, et al. Race, social class, and epidemiologic research. *Am J Epidemiol* 144: 531–536, 1996.

26. Moceri VM, et al. Early-life risk factors and the development of Alzheimer's disease. *Neurology* 54: 415–420, 2000.

27. Levy B, Langer E. Aging free from negative stereotypes: successful memory in China and among the American deaf. *J Pers Soc Psychol* 66(6): 989–997, 1994.

28. Wilson RA. *Feminine Forever*. New York: Pocket Books, 1968: 152, 35.

29. Same as 33.

30. Weissman MM, Olfson M. Depression in women: implications for health care research. *Science* 269(5225): 799–801, 1995.

31. Van Hall EV, et al. "Perimenopausal" complaints in women and men: a comparative study. *J Womens Health* 41: 45–49, 1994.

32. McKinlay J, et al. The relative contributions of endocrine changes and social circumstances to depression in mid-aged women. *J Health Soc Behav* 28(4): 345–363, 1987.

33. Schneider LS, et al. Eligibility of Alzheimer's disease clinic patients for clinical trials. *J Am Geriatr Assoc* 45: 923–938, 1997.

34. Haskell SG, et al. The effect of estrogen replacement therapy on cognitive function in women: a critical review of the literature. *J Clin Epidemiol* 50(11): 1249–1264, 1997.

35. Yaffe K, et al. Estrogen therapy in postmenopausal women—effects on cognitive function and dementia. *JAMA* 279(9): 688–695, 1998.

36. Same as 29.

37. Polo-Kantola P, et al. The effect of short-term estrogen replacement therapy on cognition: a randomized, double-blind, cross-over trial in postmenopausal women. *Obstet Gynecol* 91: 459–466, 1998.

38. Same as 28.

39. Holte A. Menopause, mood and hormone replacement therapy: methodological issues. *Maturitas* 29: 5–18, 1998.

40. Cagnacci A, et al. Effect of long-term local or systemic hormone replacement therapy on post-menopausal mood disturbances. Influences of socio-economic and personality factors. *Maturitas* 31: 111–116, 1999.

41. Polo-Kantola P, et al. When does estrogen replacement therapy improve sleep quality? *Am J Obstet Gynecol* 178: 1002–1009, 1998.

42. Owens JF, Matthews KA. Sleep disturbance in healthy middle-aged women. *Maturitas* 30: 41–50, 1998.

43. Small GW, et al. Diagnosis and treatment of Alzheimer disease and related disorders—consensus statement of the American Association for Geriatric Psychiatry, the Alzheimer's Association, and the American Geriatrics Society. *JAMA* 278(16): 1363–1371, 1997.

44. Slaven L, Lee C. Mood and symptom reporting among middle-aged women: the relationship between menopausal status, hormone replacement therapy, and exercise participation. *Health Psychol* 16(3): 203–208, 1997.

45. Pearlstein TB. Hormones and depression: what are the facts about premenstrual syndrome, menopause, and hormone replacement therapy? *Am J Obstet Gynecol* 173(2): 647–653, 1995.

46. Hunt K, et al. Mortality in a cohort of long-term users of hormone replacement therapy: an updated analysis. *Br J Obstet Gynaecol* 97: 1080–1086, 1990.

47. Breteler MMB, et al. Epidemiology of Alzheimer's disease. *Epidemiol Rev* 14: 59–82, 1992.

48. Herbert LE, et al. Is the risk of developing Alzheimer's disease greater for women than for men? *Am J Epidemiol* 153: 132–136, 2001.

49. Jorm AF. Alzheimer's disease: risk and protection. *Med J Aust* 167: 443–446, 1997.

50. Tang MX, et al. The APOE-e4 allele and the risk of Alzheimer's disease among African Americans, whites, and Hispanics. *JAMA* 279(10): 751–755, 1998.

51. Fox P. From senility to Alzheimer's disease: the rise of the Alzheimer's disease movement. *Milbank Q* 67(1): 58–102, 1989.

52. Small GW, et al. Diagnosis and treatment of Alzheimer's disease and related disorders—consensus statement of the American Association for Geriatric Psychiatry, the Alzheimer's Association, and the American Geriatrics Society. *JAMA* 278(16): 1363–1371, 1997.

53. Same as 34.

54. McCann J, et al. Why Alzheimer's disease is a women's health issue. *JAMA* 52: 132–137, 1997.

55. Shumaker SA, et al. The Women's Health Initiative Memory Study (WHIMS): a trial of the effect of estrogen therapy in preventing and slowing the progression of dementia. *Control Clin Trials* 19: 604–621, 1998.

56. Wang PN, et al. Effects of estrogen on cognition, mood, and cerebral blood flow in AD: a controlled study. *Neurology* 54(11): 2061–2066, 2000.

57. Mulnard RA, et al. Estrogen replacement therapy for treatment of mild to moderate Alzheimer's disease: a randomized controlled trial. Alzheimer's Disease Cooperative Study. *JAMA* 283(8): 1007–1015, 2000.

58. Henderson VW, et al. Estrogen for Alzheimer's disease in women: randomized, double-blind, placebo-controlled trial. *Neurology* 54(2): 295–301, 2000.

Chapter 13

1. Castelo-Branco C, et al. Skin collagen changes related to age and hormone replacement therapy. *Maturitas* 15: 113–119, 1992.

2. Savvas M, et al. Type III collagen content in the skin of post-menopausal women receiving oestradiol and testosterone implants. *Br J Obstet Gynaecol* 100(2): 154–156, 1993.

3. Haapasaari KM, et al. Systematic therapy with estrogen or estrogen with progestin has no effect on skin collagen in postmenopausal women. *Maturitas* 27: 153–162, 1997.

4. Dunn LB, et al. Does estrogen prevent skin aging? Results from the first National Health and Nutrition Examination Survey (NHANES I). *Arch Dermatol* 133: 339–342, 1997.

5. Henry F, et al. Age-related changes in facial skin contours and rheology. *J Am Geriatr Soc* 45(2): 220–222, 1997.

6. Castelo-Branco C, et al. Facial wrinkling in postmenopausal women. Effects of smoking status and hormone replacement therapy. *Maturitas* 29: 75–86, 1998.

7. Ashcroft GS, et al. Estrogen accelerates cutaneous wound healing associated with an increase in TGF-ß1 levels. *Nat Med* 3(11): 1209–1215, 1997.

8. Mor Z, Caspi E. Cutaneous complications of hormonal replacement therapy. *Clin Dermatol* 15: 147–154, 1997.

9. Graham-Brown R. Dermatologic problems of the menopause. *Clin Dermatol* 15: 143–145, 1997.

10. Fantl JA, et al. Estrogen therapy in the management of urinary incontinence in postmenopausal women: a meta-analysis. First report of the Hormones and Urogenital Therapy Committee. *Obstet Gynecol* 83(1): 12–18, 1994.

11. Sultana CJ, Walters MD. Estrogen and urinary incontinence in women. *Maturitas* 20: 129–138, 1995.

12. Jackson S. The effect of oestrogen supplementation on post-menopausal urinary stress incontinence: a double-blind placebo-controlled trial. *Br J Obstet Gynaecol* 106: 711–718, 1999.

13. Fantl JA, et al. Efficacy of estrogen supplementation in the treatment of urinary incontinence. *Obstet Gynecol* 88(5): 745–749, 1996.

14. Weinberger MW, Goodman BM, Carnes M. Long-term efficacy of nonsurgical urinary incontinence treatment in elderly women. *J Gerontol Med Sci* 54A(3): M117–M121, 1999.

15. Grady D, et al. Postmenopausal hormones and incontinence: the heart and estrogen/progestin replacement study. *Obstet Gynecol* 97: 116–120, 2001.

16. Thom DH, Van den Eeden SK, Brown JS. Evaluation of parturition and other reproductive variables as risk factors for urinary incontinence in later life. *Obstet Gynecol* 90(6): 983–989, 1997.

17. Same as 16.

18. Sand G. *Is It Hot in Here or Is It Me? A Personal Look at the Facts, Fallacies, and Feelings of Menopause.* New York: Harper Collins, 1993.

19. Brody JE. A tad of testosterone adds zest to menopause. *New York Times* February 24: C7, 1998.

20. Davis SR, et al. Testosterone enhances estradiol's effects on post-menopausal bone density and sexuality. *Maturitas* 21: 227–236, 1995.

21. Kaplan HS, Owett T. The female androgen deficiency syndrome. *J Sex Marital Ther* 19(1): 3–24, 1993.

22. Rannevik G, et al. A longitudinal study of the perimenopausal transition: altered profiles of steroid and pituitary hormones, SHBG and bone mineral density. *Maturitas* 21: 103–113, 1995.

23. Kirchengast S, et al. Decreased sexual interest and its relationship to body build in postmenopausal women. *Maturitas* 23: 63–71, 1996.

24. Bachmann GA, et al. Sexual expression and its determinants in the post-menopausal woman. *Maturitas* 6: 19–29, 1984.

25. Same as 24.

26. Hughes CL, et al. Reproductive hormone levels in gynecologic oncology patients undergoing surgical castration after spontaneous menopause. *Gynecol Oncol* 40: 42–45, 1991.

27. Casson PR, et al. Effect of postmenopausal estrogen replacement on circulating androgens. *Obstet Gynecol* 90(6): 995–998, 1997.

28. Davis SR, et al. Testosterone enhances estradiol's effects on post-menopausal bone density and sexuality. *Maturitas* 21: 227–236, 1995.

29. Same as 21.

30. Greenwood S. Testosterone supplements for women—a mixed blessing. *Network News* (National Women's Health Network) September/October: 3, 8, 1994.

31. Slayden SM. Risks of menopausal androgen supplementation. *Semin Reprod Endocrinol* 16(2): 145–152, 1998.

Chapter 15

1. Thom T, National Heart, Lung, and Blood Institute, Epidemiology Branch, personal communication, 1992.

2. Miller BA, et al., eds. *Cancer Statistics Review*, 1973–1989. National Cancer Institute, NIH publication no. 92-2789, 1992.

3. Schairer C, Lubin J, Troisi R, et al. Menopausal estrogen and estrogen-progestin replacement therapy and breast cancer risk. *JAMA* 283: 485–491, 2000.

4. The writing group for the PEPI trial. Effects of estrogen or estrogen/progestin regimens on heart disease risk factors in postmenopausal women. The Postmenopausal Estrogen/Progestin Intervention (PEPI) trial. *JAMA* 273(3): 199–208, 1995.

Chapter 16

1. Freedman RR, Woodward S. Behavioral treatment of menopausal hot flushes: evaluation by ambulatory monitoring. *Am J Obstet Gynecol* 167(2): 436–439, 1992.

2. Freedman RR, Woodward S, Brown B, Javaid JI, Pandley GN. Biochemical and thermoregulatory effects of behavioral treatment for menopausal hot flashes. *Menopause* 2: 211–218, 1995.

3. Hammar M, et al. Does physical exercise influence the frequency of postmenopausal hot flushes? *Acta Obstet Gynecol Scand* 69: 409–412, 1990.

4. Benson H, Beary JF, Carol MP. The relaxation response. *Psychiatry* 37: 37–46, 1974.

5. Irvin JH, Domar AD, Clark C, et al. The effects of relaxation response training on menopausal symptoms. *J Psychosom Obstet Gynecol* 17: 202–207, 1996.

6. Boston Women's Health Book Collective. *The New Our Bodies, Ourselves.* New York: Simon and Schuster, 1992: 406.

7. Chalker R, Whitmore KE. *Overcoming Bladder Disorders.* New York: Harper and Row, 1990.

8. Same as 7.

9. Burgio KL, Goode PS. Behavioral interventions for incontinence in ambulatory geriatric patients. *Am J Med Sci* 314: 257–261, 1997.

10. Doress PD, Siegal DL. *Ourselves, Growing Older.* New York: Simon and Schuster, 1994.

11. Love S. *Dr. Susan Love's Hormone Book.* New York: Random House, 1997.

12. Greenwood S. *Menopause, Naturally.* San Francisco: Volcano Press, 1989.

13. Voda, AM. *Menopause, Me, and You: The Sound of Women Pausing.* Binghamton, NY: Haworth Press, 1997.

14. Ito D. *Without Estrogen: Natural Remedies for Menopause and Beyond.* New York: Carol Southern Books, 1994.

15. McDowell BJ, Engberg S, Sereika S, et al. Effectiveness of behavioral therapy to treat incontinence in homebound older adults. *J Am Geriatr Soc* 47(3): 309–318, 1999.

16. Berghmans LC, Hendriks HJ, Bø K, et al. Conservative treatment of stress urinary incontinence in women: a systematic review of randomized clinical trials. *Br J Urolol* 82(2): 181–191, 1998.

17. Bø K, Talseth T, Holme I. Single-blind, randomized controlled trial of pelvic floor exercises, electrical stimulation, vaginal cones, and no treatment in management of genuine stress incontinence in women. *BMJ* 318: 487–493, 1999.

18. Cummings SR. Bone mass and bone loss in the elderly: a special case? *Int J Fertil Menopausal Stud* 38(2 suppl): 92–97, 1993.

19. Ray WA, et al. Benzodiazepines of long and short elimination half-life and the risk of hip fracture. *JAMA* 262(23): 3303–3307, 1989.

20. Liu B, et al. Use of selective serotonin-reuptake inhibitors or tricyclic antidepressants and risk of hip fractures in elderly people. *Lancet* 351: 1303–1307, 1998.

21. Tromp AM, et al. Predictors for falls and fractures in longitudinal aging study Amsterdam. *J Bone Miner Res* 13(12): 1932–1939, 1998.

22. Wolfe S. Worst pills, best pills 1999; Public Citizen Health Research Group, 1600 20th Street, NW, Washington, DC 20009.

Cited in Public Citizen Health Research Group's Health Letter 15(4): 1999.

23. Close J, et al. Prevention of Falls in the Elderly Trial (PROFET); a randomized controlled trial. *Lancet* 353: 93–97, 1999.

24. Frey C. Article to be published in *Biomechanics* 1998. Cited in Brody J. When the elderly fall, shoes may be to blame. *New York Times* February 24: C7, 1998.

25. Campbell AJ, et al. Randomized controlled trial of a general practice programme of home based exercise to prevent falls in elderly women. *BMJ* 315: 1065–1068, 1997.

26. Gregg EW, et al. Physical activity and osteoporotic fracture risk in older women. *Ann Intern Med* 129(2): 81–88, 1998.

27. Lauritzen JB, et al. Effect of external hip protectors on hip fractures. *Lancet* 341: 11–13, 1993.

28. Hinds K, Lauritzen JB. Intervention study with hip protectors (presentation). European Congress on Osteoporosis, Berlin, September 1998.

29. Padded clothing prevents life-threatening hip fractures. Elder Service Plan of the East Boston Neighborhood Health Center, November 2, 2000.

30. Kannus P, Parkkari J, Niemi S, et al. Prevention of hip fracture in elderly people with use of a hip protector. *NEJM* 343: 1506–1513, 2000.

31. Rubenstein L. Hip protectors—a breakthrough in fracture prevention. *NEJM* 343: 1562–1563, 2000.

32. Cauley JA, et al. Endogenous estrogen levels and calcium intakes in postmenopausal women. *JAMA* 260(21): 3150–3155, 1988.

33. Riis B, et al. Does calcium supplementation prevent postmenopausal bone loss? A double-blind, controlled clinical study. *NEJM* 316: 173–177, 1987.

34. Reid IR, et al. Effect of calcium supplementation on bone loss in postmenopausal women. *NEJM* 328(7): 460–464, 1993.

35. Dawson-Hughes B, et al. Effect of calcium and vitamin D supplementation on bone density in men and women 65 years of age or older. *NEJM* 337(10): 670–675, 1997.

36. Aloia JF, et al. Calcium supplementation with and without hormone replacement therapy to prevent postmenopausal bone loss. *Ann Intern Med* 120(2): 97–103, 1994.

37. Dawson-Hughes B, et al. A controlled trial of the effect of calcium supplementation on bone density in postmenopausal women. *NEJM* 323: 878–883, 1990.

38. Holbrook TL, et al. Dietary calcium and risk of hip fracture: 14-year prospective population study. *Lancet* II: 1046–1049, 1988.

39. Same as 36.

40. Meunier PJ. Prevention of hip fractures. *Am J Med* 95(5A): 75S–78S, 1993.

41. Greendale GA, et al. Lifestyle factors and bone mineral density: the postmenopausal estrogen/progestins intervention study. *J Womens Health* 4(3): 231–243, 1995.

42. Feskanich D, et al. Milk, dietary calcium, and bone fractures in women: a 12-year prospective study. *Am J Public Health* 87(6): 992–997, 1997.

43. Colditz GA, et al. The nurses' study: 20 year contribution to the understanding of health among women. *J Womens Health* 6(1): 49–62, 1997.

44. Cumming RG, Nevitt MC. Calcium for the prevention of osteoporotic fractures in postmenopausal women. *J Bone Miner Res* 12(9): 1321–1329, 1997.

45. Cummings SR, et al., for the Study of Osteoporotic Fractures Research Group. Endogenous hormones and the risk of hip and vertebral fractures among older women. *NEJM* 339(11): 733–738, 1998.

46. Chapuy MC, et al. Vitamin D and calcium to prevent hip fractures in elderly women. *NEJM* 327: 1637–1642, 1992. Cited in Cumming RG, Nevitt MC. Calcium for the prevention of osteoporotic fractures in postmenopausal women. *J Bone Miner Res* 12(9): 1321–1329, 1997.

47. Nielson FH. Studies on the relationship between boron and magnesium which possibly effects the formation and maintenance of bone. *Magnes Trace Elem* 9(2): 61–69, 1990.

48. Brown S. Osteoporosis: an anthropologist sorts facts from fallacy. Unpublished longer version of article Osteoporosis: sorting fact from fallacy. *Network News* (National Women's Health Network) July/August: 1, 5–6, 1988.

49. Campbell TC. Interview. Health Facts (Center for Medical Consumers) 22(10): 4–5, 1997.

50. Hu JF, et al. Dietary calcium and bone density among middle-aged and elderly women in China. *Am J Clin Nutr* 58: 219–227, 1993.

51. Abelow BJ, et al. Cross-cultural association between dietary animal protein and hip fracture: a hypothesis. *Calcif Tissue Int* 50(1): 14–18, 1992. Cited in Health Facts (Center for Medical Consumers) 22(10): 4–5, 1997.

52. Marsh AG, et al. Cortical bone density of adult lacto-ovo vegetarian and omnivorous women. *J Am Diet Assoc* 76: 148–151, 1980. Cited in Love S. *Dr. Susan Love's Hormone Book.* New York: Random House, 1997: 195.

53. Robbins R. *Diet for a New America.* Walpole, NH: Stillpoint Publishing, 1987.

54. Ministry of Agriculture, Fisheries and Food (UK). Manual of Nutrition (R.B. 342); Her Majesty's Stationary Office, London, 1989.

55. Wyshak G, Frish RE. Carbonated beverages, dietary calcium, the dietary calcium/phosphorus ratio, and bone fractures in girls and boys. *J Adolesc Health* 15: 210–215, 1994.

56. Kim SH, et al. Carbonated beverage consumption and bone mineral density among older women: the Rancho Bernardo study. *Am J Public Health* 87(2): 276–279, 1997.

57. Same as 56.

58. Same as 56.

59. Wyshak G, et al. Non-alcoholic carbonated beverage consumption among former college athletes. *J Orthop Res* 7: 91–99, 1989.

60. Kyro A, et al. Are smokers a risk group for delayed healing of tibial shaft fractures? *Annales Chir Gynaecol* 82(4): 254–262, 1993.

61. Baron JA. Smoking and estrogen-related disease. *Am J Epidemiol* 119(1): 9–22, 1984.

62. Same as 49.

63. Finn S. Osteoporosis: a nutritionist's approach. *Health Values* 11(4): 20–23, 1987.

64. Chow A, et al. Effect of two randomised exercise programmes on bone mass of healthy postmenopausal women. *BMJ* 295: 1441–1444, 1987.

65. Simkin A, et al. Increased trabecular bone density due to bone-loading exercises in postmenopausal osteoporotic women. *Calcif Tissue Int* 40: 59–63, 1987.

66. Zhang J, et al. Moderate physical activity and bone density among perimenopausal women. *Am J Public Health* 82(5): 736–738, 1992.

67. Danz AM, et al. The effect of a specific strength development exercise on bone mineral density in perimenopausal and postmenopausal women. *J Womens Health* 7(6): 701–709, 1998.

68. Heinonen A, et al. Randomized controlled trial of effect of high-impact exercise on selected factors for osteoporotic fractures. *Lancet* 348: 1343–1347, 1996.

69. McMurdo MET, Mole PA, Paterson CR. Controlled trial of weight bearing exercise in older women in relation to bone density and falls. *BMJ* 314: 569, 1997.

70. Greendale GA, et al. Lifestyle factors and bone mineral density: the postmenopausal estrogen/progestins intervention study. *J Womens Health* 4(3): 231–243, 1995.

71. Prince RL, et al. Prevention of postmenopausal osteoporosis: a comparative study of exercise, calcium supplementation, and hormone-replacement therapy. *NEJM* 325(17): 1189–1195, 1991.

72. Nelson ME, et al. A 1-year walking program and increased dietary calcium in postmenopausal women: effects on bone. *Am J Clin Nutr* 53: 1304–1311, 1991.

73. Nelson ME, et al. Effects of high-intensity strength training on multiple risk factors for osteoporotic fractures. *JAMA* 272(24): 1909–1914, 1994.

74. Hemingway H, Marmot M. Evidence based cardiology: psychosocial factors in the aetiology and prognosis of coronary heart disease. Systematic review of prospective cohort studies. *BMJ* 318(7196): 1460–1467, 1999.

75. Marmot MG, Bosma H, Hemingway H, et al. Contribution of job control and other risk factors to social variations in coronary heart disease incidence. *Lancet* 350(9073): 235–239, 1997.

76. Ornish D, Scherwitz LW, Billings JH, el al. Intensive lifestyle changes for reversal of coronary heart disease. *JAMA* 280(23): 2001–2007, 1998.

77. Anderson JW, Johnstone BM, Cook-Newell ME. Meta-analysis of the effects of soy protein intake on serum lipids. *NEJM* 333(5): 276–282, 1995.

78. Stampfer MJ, Hennekens CH, Manson JE, el al. Vitamin E consumption and the risk of coronary disease in women. *NEJM* 328(20): 1444–1449, 1993.

79. Stampfer MJ, Malinow MR, Willett WC, et al. A prospective study of plasma homocysteine and risk of myocardial infarction in US physicians. *JAMA* 268: 877–881, 1992.

80. Genest JJ, McNamara DN, Salem JR, et al. Plasma homocys(e)ine levels in men with premature coronary artery disease. *J Am Coll Cardiol* 16: 1114–1119, 1990.

81. Israelsson B, Brattstrom LE, Hultberg BL. Homocysteine and myocardial infarction. *Atherosclerosis* 71: 227–233, 1988.

82. Coull BM, Malinow MR, Beamer N, et al. Elevated plasma homocysteine concentration as a possible independent risk factor for stroke. *Stroke* 21: 572–576, 1990.

83. Selhub J, Jacques PF, Wilson PWF, et al. Vitamin status and intake as primary determinants of homocysteinemia in an elderly population. *JAMA* 270(22): 2693–2698.

84. Senti FR, Pilch SM. Analysis of folate data from the second Nutritional Health and Nutrition Examination Survey (NHANES). *J Nutr* 115: 1398–1402, 1985.

85. Eaton CB, Menard LM. A systematic review of physical activity promotion in primary care office settings. *Br J Sports Med* 32: 11–16, 1998.

86. Andersen RE, Crespo CJ, Bartlett SJ, Cheskin LJ, Pratt M. Relationship of physical activity and television watching with body weight and level of fatness among children: results from the third National Health and Nutrition Examination Survey. *JAMA* 279: 938–942, 1998.

87. Same as 85.

88. Pate RR, Pratt M, Blair SN, et al. Physical activity and public health: a recommendation from the Centers of Disease Control and Prevention and the American College of Sports Medicine. *JAMA* 273: 402–407, 1995.

89. Fiatarone MA, Marks EC, Ryan ND, et al. High-intensity training in nonagenarians: effects of skeletal muscle. *JAMA* 263: 3029–3034, 1990.

Index

Please note: The abbreviations ERT and HRT are used to denote estrogen replacement therapy and hormone replacement therapy, respectively.